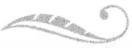

Praise for **Riding Horseback in Purple**

"Alice MacGillivray has done us all a great favor by writing
Riding Horseback in Purple: She has given us the exhortation to
follow our passion for horses but tempered it with some of
the soundest and most sage advice about how to do it. This
book should become the bible for those wonderfully enthu-
siastic middle-aged souls who are pondering whether to
return to their life-long passion for horses and finally making the jump to owning a horse of their own!"

ALLAN J. HAMILTON, MD, Professor of Neurosurgery and author
of *Zen Mind, Zen Horse*

"A MUST read for ANYONE considering purchasing a horse.
With its logical, practical and useful tidbits it will truly set
you up for success! It also proves that dreams do come true!"

PATTI JO WALTER, owner/operator of Francis Creek Fjords

"Amazingly well thought out and researched. Alice speaks
directly from experience and with a sense of humour, which
I feel is essential in this horse world. This book is perfect
for the beginner equestrian starting down the path of horse
ownership."

DEBORAH M. FOX, Equine Canada dressage coach and dressage judge

"The author's journey from total newbie to full-fledged equestrian and horse owner is chronicled with wisdom, insight, and humour. This engaging book lights the way for other mature women who are hoping to realize their own equestrian dream, while avoiding the pitfalls. A useful and practical guide, with a touch of the mystical that horses bring into our lives."

LORI ALBROUGH, Bluebird Lane Fjords

"People used to have direct experience with large animals by growing up on farms; now they start from scratch. This book offers a big step towards better understanding the modern world of horses through knowledge and mindful awareness, leading to healthy and comfortable daily interactions with our beloved equines."

PHILLIP ODDEN, owner, Fjord Farm and Norsk Wood Works Ltd.

"This is not just a story about one woman's transformational ascent to horse ownership, rather this is a story of great significance to us all in a human-built world. It's an honest conversation about the realities of owning a horse, how to lean into that experience, and the deep and committed tending of the soul we need in the world. This book is a story of 're-membering' our compartmentalized bodies into whole and ancient selves through a cultivated bond between humans and horses."

JEFF LEINAWEAVER, PhD, Graduate Faculty in Sustainability, Bainbridge Graduate Institute

ALICE E. MACGILLIVRAY, PhD

Riding Horseback in Purple

Re-awakening the Dream of Owning a Horse

14 15 16 17 18   5 4 3 2 1

Gabriola Island
British Columbia, Canada
www.4KM.net

Library and Archives Canada Cataloguing in Publication

MacGillivray, Alice, 1952–, author
Riding horseback in purple : reawakening the dream
of owning a horse / Alice MacGillivray.
Includes bibliographical references and index.
Issued in print and electronic formats.

ISBN 978-0-9936151-0-8 (pbk.)
ISBN 978-0-9936151-1-5 (ebook)

1. Horses--Behavior. 2. Horses--Training.
3. Women horse owners. I. Title.
SF285.3.M34 2014   636.1'3   C2013-907890-8
C2013-907891-6

Editing by Barbara Pulling
Copy editing by Shirarose Wilensky
Index by Annette Lorek
Cover and text design by Jessica Sullivan
Cover photograph by Bob Langrish

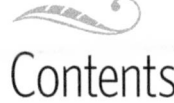

Contents

||||||||||||||||||||

Introduction

THE TITLE OF *Riding Horseback in Purple* is inspired by the first line of Jenny Joseph's cheerfully rebellious poem, "Warning": "When I am an old woman I shall wear purple." This book is written for women, like me, who are somewhat near what they think of as "retirement age" and are revisiting the dream that wouldn't go away: the dream of owning a horse. I have gotten to know so many women in their forties, fifties, sixties, and seventies who have horses in their lives, often after a long period of time when they had other priorities. I have also heard many adult women say things like "I had not intended to buy a project," when they realized their horse wasn't the best one they could have chosen for this stage of their life. And I have heard horse experts talk about women who finally get a horse and a couple of years later are searching for a new owner. I want to help women connect with great horses so that they can grow, learn, and enjoy active lives as partners with their horses.

I have a beautiful Norwegian Fjord mare named Bocina, born in Pennsylvania, raised and trained in Ontario, and now living here on Gabriola Island on the west coast of Canada. She was nine when I bought her, and I was in my fifties. She is my first and only horse. In some respects, I am a typical Canadian horse owner: a woman in my fifties with some university education. In other respects, I am beating the odds. I keep hearing about new horse owners who gave up quickly. I have never considered parting with Bocina, but I have built a strong foundation of knowledge, friends—online and in person—and emotional commitment that have helped me through a few fragile times. If I had not learned some of the things I share in this book, I might have given up.

Giving up has many layers. I consider it a tragedy when a potentially great horsewoman gives up a potentially great horse partner because she is not well prepared and doesn't know how to close that gap. It is equally sad to see a woman who takes on a horse by herself, cannot problem solve on her own, and gives up without finding a community. This isolation may leave the woman feeling unsuccessful and the horse feeling vulnerable.

It was not long ago that horses were a huge part of our lives. As a young child living in an old-fashioned neighbourhood, I recall watching the milk delivery horse with fascination. He knew exactly where to stop and stood like a rock as the milkman jogged up to the little milk box doors on the sides of the brick houses. Sometimes, the milkman would put the horse's feed bag on across from our house, which added to the excitement for an animal-crazy kid. On rare occasions, I saw horses ploughing fields. Many of our great-grandparents relied primarily on horses to carry out day-to-day activities. They probably thought of the human-horse relationships in very practical terms. Yet consider how much they learned about how to treat other beings firmly but kindly, how to learn from mistakes, and how to communicate with a very different species. How did that experience influence other aspects of their lives? How did it affect their independence? What would happen to us today if gas pumps closed, for example? Imagine trying to explain our extreme reliance on disappearing fossil fuels to an ancestor who travelled on horseback and by horse and carriage. I asked one of the women I interviewed for this book what we would lose if we no longer had horses, and she replied succinctly: "Our American heritage."

To this book, I bring my intense learning about horse ownership from the last few years. Yet many other aspects of my life contribute as well. I have always loved animals and was a veterinary assistant as a young adult. I only worked with small animals, but those experiences fine-tuned my observational skills. I became good at noticing small nuances of body language and helping animals to gain even a little trust in a stressful environment. When I was told "women can't get into veterinary college, especially for large animals" (how things have changed), I became a certified professional dog groomer so that I could spend more time with animals outside my home. Long after I gave up my shop, I would go to retired people's homes, as some had a lot of difficulty driving into cities to a grooming shop. This was more of a community service than a business, and I really enjoyed it. I often think back to a Scottie owned by a relaxed elderly couple in a trailer park. They said no one else had been able to groom Tammy, because the groomers and Tammy got into "big fights" and the groomers said she was dangerous. There wasn't a dangerous bone in that dog's body. She talked by growling. I loved going to groom her. We'd have growling conversations and, as she was young and very energetic, I'd let her off the table every fifteen minutes or so to play. The old couple would sit in their living room methodically completing a crossword puzzle while Tammy roared up and down the trailer with a braided rope toy in her powerful jaws, getting traction and speed on the carpet and sliding to bumpy stops on the linoleum. I'd scoop her up again, cuddle her and do the next stage. I think she enjoyed my visits as much as I did. Decades later, I wonder how Tammy fared when I moved to another part of the country. You might think that all this practice with dogs (and cats) put me in a great position to communicate with horses. But I sheepishly admit it didn't help as much as I had hoped. My body language skills helped me to see that "something" was being communicated, but I was much less certain of what.

Later in life, I worked for many years with large park organizations, where I helped manage the relationships among habitat, wildlife, visitors, facilities, safety and quality of experience. I was encouraged to join parks because I had spent a lot of time outdoors and knew a lot about natural history. Although things like species identification got me through that first interview, my most important lesson was about how different life forms are connected. Fungi influence trees (often in positive ways), trees influence birds, birds influence the spread of understory plants, and so on. Humans are rapidly forgetting the many ways in which they can and should connect with natural environments. It is amazing that horses will allow desensitized lifelong urban dwellers to come near them, let alone climb on their backs.

Another thread that weaves through my education and career has been about how adults learn and how we develop, share, and use our knowledge. Although I work in formal education, I am the first to admit that most learning happens through life experience. The island where I now live is a study in experiential learning. People are always helping others learn about everything from contra dancing to geothermal power generation. Many residents are retired, but few seem to be quietly retired. They publish and act and sing and lobby government and design new governance structures well into their eighties and nineties. Learning and activity (horses clearly make us do both) can promote health and longevity.

Having a horse is both an adventure and a commitment to lifelong learning. I was a rebellious adventurer who did many things early in life (such as moving to the West Coast alone at sixteen), and I learned many other things late in life (I got my undergraduate degree and an MA in leadership in my forties, and an MA in human development and a PhD in systems in my fifties). Much of my consulting work has been in the field of leadership. Because the work we do with horses is always about leadership, the leadership connection has been an especially rich one for me.

Finally, I believe writing is a way of both teaching and learning: learning about the subject matter, learning about people, learning about yourself, and trying to share in ways that will make a difference in other people's lives. Over the years, I have written newspaper columns about nature, environmental education materials for schools, and academic papers. But none felt as important as this book.

This book focuses on information I had difficulty finding as I went through the process of selecting, buying, and learning to work with my first horse. At times, the information was out there but not presented in ways that helped me understand its importance or context. Sometimes good information was out there, but I hadn't yet developed the network through which I could find good authors and coaches when I was ready for them. There are many excellent specialized books and DVDs about everything from designing your property layout for accommodating a horse to learning to ride. I touch on such subjects and reference other authors who might be helpful for you.

Riding Horseback in Purple has two sections. The first section helps you to decide whether this is the time to get your horse, how to shop for the right horse, and how to prepare effectively for your horse's arrival. Here, I explore the knowledge, skills, equipment, and resources you will need. I share stories from my experience, reference experts, and include tools such as checklists. There are key "points to ponder" and a "question to consider" at the end of each chapter.

The second section focuses on what to do after your horse arrives. For example, how do you deal with the changes in diet that may happen when your horse is in a new location? I address common errors and misconceptions associated with day-to-day management. This section explores the building relationship between you and your horse. There is no recipe book for this. Each horse is unique; each person is unique. As a matter of fact, each day and each encounter with your horse is different. There are other in-depth books by experts about connecting with horses. What I bring is insight into the learning curve, the questions you face, and the challenges of learning for a novice without decades of experience interacting with horses. This section will be most meaningful as you start to work with your horse. You may want to come back to it over time as your expertise grows and new questions come to mind. Again, each chapter ends with points to ponder.

I want to comment on terminology in this book. I alternate the use of pronouns for horses ("him," "her"), because I am sometimes referring to a specific male or female horse, and so that no one feels ignored through the whole book if they only have a mare or a gelding. I also use terms such as "who" instead of "that" or "which." I grew up in a time when it was practically a sin to anthropomorphize: to attribute human characteristics to a non-human animal. But times are changing. Our old rules about what makes humans unique (tool use, language, and so on) keep crumbling. And scientists are learning more about the emotions and abilities of animals. So I would rather err on the side of respectful common ground than adhere to the idea of humans being totally different (and presumably much better) than other animals. I occasionally use words that might seem academic or like jargon. I know different readers will have different reactions, but I hope this is a way of opening doors to other learning by introducing common terms in related fields.

They say it takes a village to raise a child. It also takes a community to nurture the growth of a novice horsewoman. You may be on the verge of joining a network—larger and more fascinating than you can imagine—where people are passionate about horse health, horse behaviour, safety of horsewomen, horses and empowerment, horses and leadership, positive aging, dressage, pleasure riding, natural horsemanship, horse-human communication, horse rescue, and dozens of other facets of life with horses. Join me for some glimpses into these explorations.

||||||||||||||||||||

Acknowledgements

FIRST, A BIG THANK YOU to everyone in the Gabriola Island horse community, an amazing group of people (you know who you are) who care about their horses, their learning, and their community. Bocina thanks you, too, for everything from places to call home through games of hoofball to behind-the-ear scratches.

A special thanks to Patti Jo Walter, the renowned matchmaker from Francis Creek Fjords in the American Midwest. Patti Jo confirmed from a distance—with her deep knowledge of the Fjord breed—that I had finally intuited my way to the "right horse." She listened to me, read about and watched videos of prospects, and made me feel totally confident with my first choice.

Barbara Pulling and Shirarose Wilensky provided excellent comments: I think the more skilled you become as a writer, the more you realize you need editors. Thank you to Jessica Sullivan, who brought magical skills to the design.

Some of the experts I reference generously made the time to review sections of the book for accuracy and to add content. A special thank you to biologist Rupert Sheldrake, whose work I have admired for decades and who reviewed a section despite his extremely busy schedule.

It was valuable to have skilled horsewomen from other parts of the continent with varied backgrounds and styles read the book for accuracy and to offer input related to their years of helping new owners. These included Lori Albrough of Bluebird Lane Fjords in Ontario, and Sandy McMahon in British Columbia.

Others connected with me from a distance through our common interests in Fjords or horses in general. Online forums have been incredibly helpful. The members' insights and stories bring important content to life and add depth that simply cannot be conveyed through factual text. Thank you to Ellen Barry; Wendy Bauwens; Holly Brewer; Claudia Cavanaugh; Robin Churchill; Brenda Fehr from Dare to Dream Horse Rescue; Jim Fiorini; Brandy Gonzalez; Pat Holland; Sharen Howarth; Julie from New Mexico; Heike Lewandowski; Corinne Logan; Sandra McCartt; Jean Nock; Phil Odden; Yvonne Olson; Sharon Quarrington; Mel Raven; Barb Renico; Paul Sherland; Fran Severn; Kay Van Natta; June Mendoza Wheeler from Saint Paul, Minnesota, Pat Wolfe, and many others.

My family isn't a horsey family, but they get an A-plus for accepting the fact I had to realize my dream, regardless of time, effort, cost, and the amount of laundry.

I need to acknowledge a few of the many women who have led the way through their research, writing, and publications. Some have inspired me through their scholarship and humanity about kind, feminine ways of understanding the world. They include Sandra Harding and Donna Haraway.

Others have generously shared their deep expertise in specific aspects of work with horses through their books. Carol Rivoire helped a lot of us learn about Fjords through her Fjordhorse Handbook. And Sally Swift, Linda Tellington-Jones, Linda Kohanov, Carolyn Resnick and Jane Savoie have all inspired me in unique ways. Thank you.

Finally, I want to acknowledge one of the many horses who have inspired me. As you learn about a breed, you learn about some of the stellar horses who exemplify good conformation, performance and temperaments. Prisco, an imported Dutch Fjord stallion (often called Dutch or Dutchie) was one of those horses for me. Simply seeing pictures of him and reading about him on the web was a big part of my growing love for the breed over the years. I didn't set out to get one of Prisco's foals, but it was a wonderful coincidence that I did. After relatively minor surgery, Dutch tragically died from rare complications. As I write this, even people who only knew of him are mourning his loss. Prisco's owner, Peggy Peregrine Spear happened to notice on a Disney studio clip that Dutch was the visual inspiration for the Fjord in the film Frozen. Hopefully they appreciated the power and presence of the horse as much as the opportunity to create a cute character.

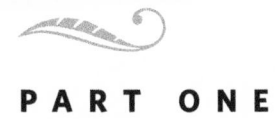

PART ONE

The Dream

Exploring and Building Readiness

WE TALK ABOUT dreams in different ways. A horse in a dream may seem as real as a horse in a pasture, yet we say the dream isn't real. A daydream or a fantasy of owning a horse may seem compelling, yet a daydream does not require care and feeding. The human mind constantly plays with ideas, memories, hopes, and reality. But there are crucial differences among them. Those of us who are parents probably wanted to be the best parents ever, yet we fell short of that goal (if not flat on our faces from time to time). So in Part I of this book, I want to acknowledge the beauty and power of the dream of owning a horse. And I also want to bring you down to earth to truly examine whether you want a dream or whether you want a horse. I map out a path for exploring and building your readiness in the hope that if you do take the plunge, you are entering into a healthy, safe, rewarding, long-term partnership with your equine companion.

The wind of heaven is that which
blows between a horse's ears.

ARABIAN PROVERB

1 | The Dream That Would Not Go Away

I RECENTLY SHARED a taxi with a gregarious twentysomething. He had asked about my broken shoulder. "So were you one of those thirteen-year-olds who was obsessed by horses and drew pictures of them?" he asked. "You have me pegged," I admitted. (It turns out he did the same thing with dolphins.) At the time, my arm was in a sling as I recovered from a surgery to repair several fractures. Yes, it was horse-related: my horse started to bolt when I was in front of her and sent me flying. No, it didn't put me off horses or horse ownership or horseback riding. And yes, I will share more of the story later, in the chapter on fear and courage.

Even before I touched a horse or rode one, I was drawn to the human-horse connection. I saved my small childhood allowance for a horse newsletter (back in hard-copy, snail-mail days). I asked for horse figurines for my birthday and Christmas. I memorized a bran mash recipe at the school library.

But my parents could not afford a horse. They did manage to pay for a few riding lessons, which were primarily trail rides. The only vaguely technical things I was taught were to keep my heels down, where the reins should thread through my fingers, and where to position my thumbs to jump over small obstacles. Boots—a sturdy black-and-white Paint—dutifully followed the horse in front of her (with one memorable exception, my only galloping experience to date), so I gained a false sense of confidence and elation about becoming a decent rider.

I spent teenage summers standing on fence rails watching horses, and I occasionally talked my way into riding them. I even got to ride in the local village parade, which was madness considering Joe wasn't very well trained and there was a steam whistle in the parade that had caused a Shetland pony to faint on several occasions. The horse field was about an hour's walk from our cottage. Occasionally, the horses were in a barn en route, only about ten minutes walk from the cottage. So I learned to whinny well enough that they would answer from the barn, saving me a couple of hours and the disappointment of arriving at an empty field. I took this whinnying ability far too seriously, thinking it signified some deep bond—or at least the ability to communicate across species boundaries.

As my life evolved, there were other interests that connected indirectly with horses. I was drawn to animals of every type (spiders being a notable exception). Neighbours had a Welsh corgi who had been abused by the child of a previous owner. At first I would just sit on the lawn near their fence, sometimes for an hour, to let Bracken know I was no threat. It took months for her to allow me to touch her, and even more time before she was eager to see me. I was fascinated by communication across species and felt privileged when an animal wanted to be in my company. Horrified by the idea that humans would deliberately mistreat animals, I raised funds for the Humane Society. As an adult, it was disturbing to hear about "unintentional" mistreatment. Were purebred dogs suffering from unexpected consequences of breeding programs? Purebred horses? Were horses stressed by dressage? Some researchers made these claims. If I ever got a horse, should I avoid purebred horses and dressage?

I wrestled with many questions over many years before taking the wonderful plunge into horse ownership. In that process, I have connected with women around my age who have stories similar to mine. Some had a practical bent: "I dream of being able to hop on a well-behaved horse after work to go for a trail ride." Some dreamt of a deep cross-species bond. Others talked about a horse as therapy, to mitigate a stressful job or relationship. Several had faced a life crisis and realized they must toss aside obstacles and return to their passions. Many had ridden extensively as teens, a few had owned horses in the past, and others were novices like me. But they were all women with considerable life experience who had shifted priorities to live more of their lives in treasured equine company.

Canada's most recent horse census data researches "industry participants" who own, care for, ride, and drive horses. The census staff members go to places such as breed registries to find people to interview so that their sample may focus more on "serious" horse people who compete, coach, and breed than on those who have lone unregistered horses in their yards. But the numbers are interesting. Participation has shifted from youth to adults. In Canada, about

60 percent of horse owners are adults, and in some parts of the country it is as high as 85 percent. A "typical participant" is a female, Internet-using baby boomer (age fifty to fifty-nine) with some post-secondary education and several pets. The oldest age category is "over 70," which includes 7 percent of participants.

I correspond with several women who participate in two small online horse forums. These forums focus on the Norwegian Fjord breed, but members often own other breeds of horses as well. When I asked them if they got their first horse (or first horse since childhood) as a mature woman, almost forty women said they did. I regularly draw on their perspectives and those of other women I have interviewed for this book. I hope our collective insights help you with your planning and choices—or at least provide some interesting entertainment.

POINTS TO PONDER

- In some parts of the world, mature female horse owners are actually typical horse owners.
- Many women who dreamt of a life with horses found that the day-to-day responsibilities of life got in the way. Yet the dream did not die.
- It is not unusual for a woman to get her first horse, or her first horse in decades, around retirement age.

QUESTION TO CONSIDER

- Why are you drawn to horses or horse ownership?

But maybe I ought to practice a little now?
So people who know me are not too shocked and surprised
When suddenly I am old, and start to wear purple.
JENNY JOSEPH

2 | White Wine and Carrots: On Being a Mature Horsewoman

THERE IS A POEM by an unknown author about her love of horses later in life that includes the line: "I shall spend my social security on white wine and carrots." As you start to muse aloud about getting a horse, people may ask: "This is your FIRST horse? Aren't you a bit...late to start?"

In a way, I envy the children who melted into horses' backs as toddlers, galloped fearlessly as children, and knew the difference between long reins and side reins as teens. Yet I value the layers of learning I have been forced to do as a result of buying a horse later in life. My friend Bonnie—who has been riding my mare, Bocina, recently—put it very well:

I've always thought it was important for us adult people to be learning new things: not to be those know-it-all complacent adults. I get lazy at this, but working with

Bocina—and now taking riding lessons—is like that. It hearkens back to time spent on horseback in my youth, yet I'm doing and learning something new.

Bonnie was talking, in part, about the brain training of continuous learning—like doing crosswords, Sudoku, or online memory games but a lot more fun for horse lovers. Research shows there can be cognitive, emotional, psychological, physical, and what some people think of as spiritual benefits to spending time with horses. As just one example, in speaking of benefits for the "over-fifty crowd," Naomi Scott describes how going for a walk on horseback gently exercises hundreds of bones and muscles. In *Special Needs, Special Horses: A Guide to the Benefits of Therapeutic Riding*, she writes: "This helps to increase fitness, balance and flexibility, encourages better posture and leads to better functioning of the cardio-vascular system." These cognitive, emotional, and physical benefits are key elements of maintaining quality of life and independence. Such benefits come almost automatically with horse ownership, but some owners take a more proactive approach.

Internet marketer and part-time horseman Paul Sherland told me about recovering from an injury. His work with computers means he needs to put effort into getting fit. To recover from his injury, he used a goal and milestones. The goal was a three-day horsemanship and cow-working clinic several months down the road. These are some of the strategies he used:

> I changed my diet, lost 15 pounds, and embarked on a program of weight lifting and aerobic exercise. During the clinic, I was one of folks who could mount without a mounting block although I was probably the

oldest member of the class (age 62) riding one of the taller horses. That fitness improved my riding and my confidence throughout the clinic.

Lori Albrough had a similar experience but took a different approach. She had learned of the "word of the year" concept. Rather than create and ignore a list of New Year's resolutions, you choose a single word for focus. Lori decided to try it. Much to her surprise, the word that came to her was "athlete." She thought of her horses as athletes. She respected the work of athletes. But this was definitely not part of her self-image. She blogged about the experience at bluebirdlane. com/my-word-of-the-year.html. I witnessed a week of Lori's efforts as an athlete and can attest to the fact that she has a very high level of fitness, which she says has influenced her horsemanship and other aspects of her life.

As I write this, I am looking at a photograph in the book *Yoga for Equestrians: A New Path for Achieving Union with the Horse*. It isn't a great photo technically, but the content is quite wonderful. Three women are in identical yoga poses on a deck (presumably of one of their homes). Because of this non-commercial setting, it seems they are friends. At least one is wearing stretchy riding pants. One—perhaps the home-owner—has a white cat standing between her feet, happy to be part of the activity. Because they are featured in this book, they are doing yoga both for their own health and to build balance and connection with horses. How wonderful is that?

If such benefits intrigue you, how might you get started?

One Route to Visibility

Most people who become horse owners start by experiencing aspects of horse ownership without the full range of responsibilities. The Canadian census describes this large group as the "invisible sector." They are participants in the horse community or industry who cannot be reached easily through standard industry communications channels. They might ride a friend's horse or take lessons at a stable.

I was one of about 300,000 Canadians in this category for a few months before buying Bocina. I looked through the Yellow Pages, guessed at a good stable for lessons, and signed up. My experience at this stable was brief but educational. Had I ever cleaned hoofs before or after my lessons as a teen? I don't think so. I had definitely never been close to horse blankets (i.e., the coats that cover horses from chest to rump to protect them from the elements). At first, it was so confusing to remember which buckles to do up or undo first. Now, it is second nature. If a horse were to take off partway through the blanketing or un-blanketing procedure, the last thing you'd want would be a panicked horse, perpetually spooked by a blanket dragging on the ground behind him. So the front of the blanket is done up first and undone last.

At the stable they asked, "You're not a timid rider, are you?" How are you supposed to answer that after more than four decades out of a saddle? "I don't think so," I replied. So I was directed to a very big gelding whom I had seen jumping something very tall in the stable's promotional materials.

One day, I went to loop the reins over a fence rail in the ring and was quickly reprimanded by the coach: "You NEVER do that!" Apparently, one of the key procedures I had garnered from Hollywood Westerns was deeply flawed. In the movies, the horses had been trained to "ground tie," or not move when the reins are dropped. Also, Western riders use split reins, which are less likely to tangle around the feet than looped reins. But some consider the practice inappropriate under any circumstances.

As I rode the big gelding, I had difficulty getting him to move into one corner of the rectangular ring. Of course, this was partly because of my rudimentary skills. When I did convince him not to cut the corner, his stride would feel uncomfortably bouncy (using my terms of that period) as we rode down the following length. I mentioned this to the coach. "Oh, that's because they used to be able to see pigs from there. They all do it," she explained. "How long ago was that?" I inquired. After a pause she replied, "About ten years." Horses have superb memories, especially if they are linked to fear. And for some reason, pigs are scary.

It was the rainy season on the North American west coast, and after a few lessons, I switched to a stable with a covered arena. I was able to compare everything from communication styles to horse care routines to the footing in the paddocks. At the new stable, the waterproof labels on each stall and paddock fascinated me. They showed what every horse was fed for each of several daily feedings. Even a small thing like this was a springboard for learning about the nutritional needs of different breeds and individual horses.

At this second stable, I saw visits by the vet and farrier, a specialist in equine hoof care, and had a good conversation with the farrier about training expectations and credentials in different countries. I watched an employee mixing feed supplements. I saw people come in for lessons and watched an equine chiropractor rehabilitate a gelding once destined to be euthanized. Everything I observed was fascinating. One day, my coach, Diana Lewall, said: "I am often surprised by how little some full-board horse owners know about horses and horse care." That was a huge eye-opener for me—and a confidence builder in preparation for my subsequent learning curves.

If you are not sure whether you want a horse, I suggest you shift the dream temporarily from owning a horse to spending time with horses. Of course it isn't the same as having your own horse. But it is a bit like training for an athletic event or a vacation with lots of hiking. You will learn a lot, build skills, have time to reflect on the realities of horse ownership, and you will be much better prepared to be a great horse owner if that day ever comes.

As you learn, strike a balance between staying open to new ideas and starting to trust your intuition about what is right for you. Don't restrict your time to *doing*; also focus on *being*. Both can help you learn, grow, and make wise decisions as you focus on finding the right horse.

POINTS TO PONDER

▸ Do not accept people's opinions that you are too late to start spending time with horses; figure that out for yourself. (You might think of clever, assertive things to say in response.)

▸ Your work with horses can result in cognitive, emotional, psychological, social, physical, and spiritual benefits.

▸ Begin on the fringes of horse ownership—taking riding lessons, for example—to determine whether you are experiencing a dream or nostalgia.

▸ Ask lots of questions. Learn everything you can from your experiences on the fringe, using both observation and intuition. This might involve some un-learning!

QUESTION TO CONSIDER

▸ What are three practical approaches that would help you learn more about horses as you move towards making your decision about ownership?

*"Some people care too much.
I think it's called love."*

A.A. MILNE

3 | Begin Your Search for the "Right" Horse

*"Forget pretty, forget connection, forget dreaming of riding
a dressage test in top hat and tails. Get the solid older
horse who has seen it all, in good health with no serious
health problems or behavior quirks. A 4H horse that
has been ridden by a younger child for several years has
usually been loved, cared for, wallowed on, been in arenas
and outside and is trustworthy."*—SANDRA MCCARTT,
executive recruiter and horsewoman

PEOPLE TALK ABOUT common mistakes of
horse purchasing. In my limited experience, most mature
women thoughtfully research and reflect before buying a
horse. They bring many years of experience from their homes
and workplaces, where they have learned about patience,
analysis, unpredictability, and impacts of choices. They are
unlikely to fall in love with—and purchase—the first hot
mare they view, just because of her beautiful eyes and flow-
ing mane (although I have learned through writing this book

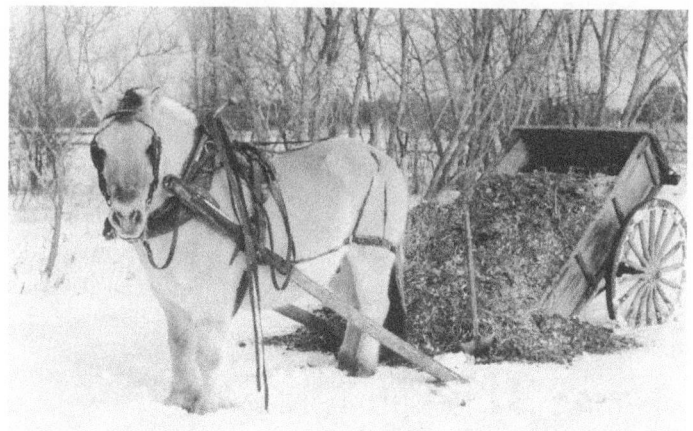

ABOVE *Even when something goes seriously wrong, well-trained Fjords like Ralph will work with you. Ralph waited while Pat went to the house to get his camera for this shot.* Photo: PAT WOLFE

that many prospective horse owners do make very question-able decisions, and I address that in more detail later in the section about risk in chapter 10 and in the afterword). I thank horsewoman Holly Brewer for helping me make sense of this paradox!

Desirable Characteristics

When I talk with mature female horse owners I know, I see four common patterns in what they are looking for:

A reliable horse. Many women look for a horse that is rela-tively unlikely to bolt, spook, or demand a huge amount of attention and skill in order to enjoy a pleasant trail ride (or even to stay in the saddle). Of course, any horse can spook or bolt, and we need to be safety conscious at all times.

A smaller horse. My mare is 14.2 hands. A hand is a unit of measure of four inches, and the height of a horse is measured

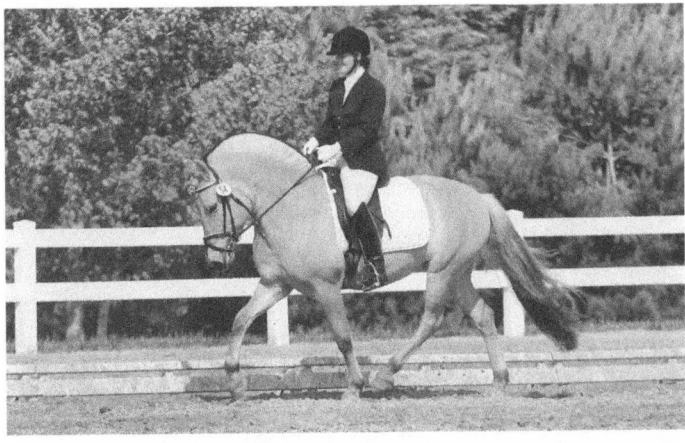

ABOVE *Lori Albrough on Kestrel. Lori is about 5'2" and Kestrel is 14 hands. Kestrel was the Grand Champion Mare at the Norwegian Fjord Horse Registry 25th Anniversary Show in Winona, Minnesota.* Photo: BLUEBIRD LANE FJORDS

from the ground to the withers at the base of the neck. Several women with beautiful larger horses have said they are envious. Few fifteen-year-old girls would crave a 14.2 horse, but as our bodies get less flexible and bounce-able as we age, a smaller horse starts to look really good.

A versatile horse. Especially with a first horse, or a first horse in decades, we may not be quite sure what we would like to do over many years of horse ownership. Trail ride? Backcountry trips? Dressage? Jumping? Driving? Helping with physical work on a rural property? We're not going to become Olympic competitors, so a breed that can do many things might be more attractive and practical than a more specialized breed.

A horse interested in bonding. Many horses are interested in a relationship for reasons we may never understand, but some will be friendlier, more inquisitive, and more inclined to bond

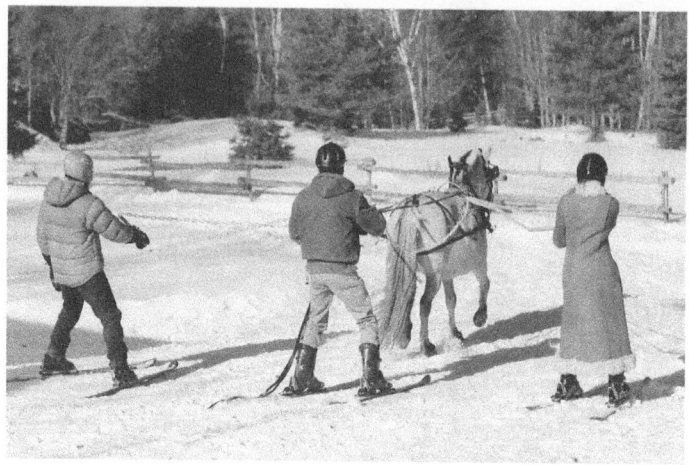

ABOVE *Pat Wolfe skijoring with friends behind Emmeline.* Photo: JANE BEALL

with you. This is not easy to predict, as it can depend on the horse's breed, history with people, age, temperament, gender, your level of confidence, and the chemistry between you.

IT IS HELPFUL to understand the different groups of breeds in relation to these four desirable characteristics, and to understand specifics about one or more of the breeds you are drawn to.

Groups of Breeds: Consider the Warm-Blooded Breeds

Horses are often categorized as hot, warm, or cold-blooded. You might have to do some searching on the web or at the library to find out in which category a particular breed belongs. These categories speak to horses' temperaments and origins and have nothing to do with blood temperature. I have heard many people talk about "warmbloods" and advertise their horses for sale as "warmbloods" (even if that is not

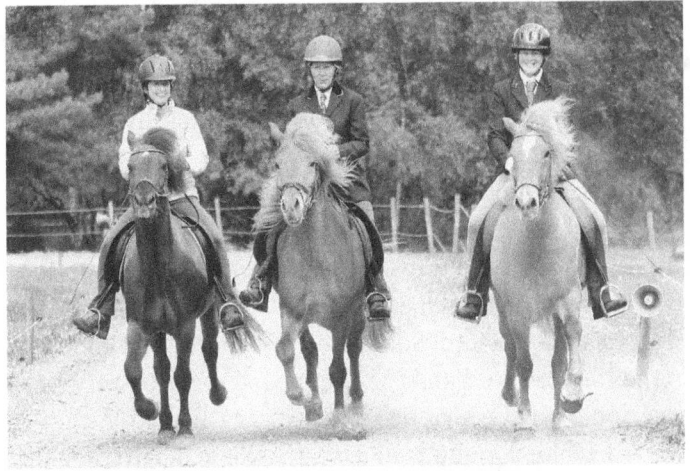

ABOVE Riding gaited Icelandic Horses in West Wales UK (solva-icelandics. co.uk) where they warn Icelandics are addictive! Icelandics are usually between 12.3 and 14.2 hands high. Photo: MIC RUSHEN

a formal part of the breed name, such as "Dutch Warmblood," for example). So far, I have never heard anyone announce: "I have a hotblood" or "I want to sell my coldblood." They are much more inclined to say: "I have an Arab stallion" (in the hotblood category) or "my Percheron mare is for sale" (in the coldblood category).

Hot-blooded horses such as Thoroughbreds and Arabians have spirit, which makes them ideal for purposes such as racing. They will rarely be good matches for the person seeking a calm, reliable horse. But there are exceptions.

Cold-blooded horses such as Clydesdales and Belgians won't fit the "smaller horse" criterion, but don't write them off because of their mass. They are sometimes called gentle giants. I have connected with women who have draft horse crosses and love them. Some sources caution that as your confidence grows, you may want more spirit in your horse. However, you might want a very quiet horse for a few years. Or you might find a heavy horse with just the right amount of spirit. As with all horses, research carefully to find a good match.

Yes, warm-blooded horses fall between hot and cold. More than sixty breeds are considered warmbloods, and many of these have a mix of breeds in their history. A few examples of warmbloods are the American Paint Horse, the Morgan, and the Norwegian Fjord. Some are very large (the Oldenburg stands between 16.2 and 17.2 hands), and some are very small (Icelandic horses may be fewer than 13 hands). Although the warmblood group is diverse, the general pattern is that warmbloods will be better suited to novices or older riders than hot-blooded breeds and will be more "forward" or energetic than cold-blooded breeds. Some of the warmbloods are gaited. In other words, they have one or more additional gaits beyond the walk, trot, and canter ridden with other breeds. Icelandics are very easy to ride, but horsemen and women spend lifetimes learning to ride them extremely well.

Norwegian Fjords as One Specific Breed to Consider

A recent study by Barbara Wallner from the University of Veterinary Medicine in Vienna explored the male ancestry of horses (a Y chromosome study). The research revealed a kind of modern horse family tree with six different lines or branches. The first was distributed widely across large geographic areas and almost all breeds. The second was similarly widespread except for some northern breeds and ones on the Iberian Peninsula. The third was common in Thoroughbreds and many warmbloods. The remaining three were distinctive breed-related lines: one in the Shetland pony, one in the

Icelandic horse, and one in the Norwegian Fjord. Fjords really are different. They are often positioned as a great breed for women introducing, or reintroducing, horses into their lives. There are good reasons for this—and some cautions as well.

I might have been able to keep my horse ownership dream dormant if it hadn't been for the Fjord breed. Something just clicked for me, and Fjords became a bit of an obsession. I love fall fairs and have always headed to the horse barns first, walking up and down the isles, curious about what I will see and the energy I will feel. I remember walking as a small child behind the standing stalls of the heavy horses at the Royal Agricultural Winter Fair in Toronto. The horses would usually be resting, so I could clearly see the plate-sized horseshoes on their upturned hooves. I must have amused the adults as I slowly walked by sideways, giving the horses a wide berth, with my eyes glued on those feet. Decades later, when I discovered the Fjord breed in the 1980s, I admit that

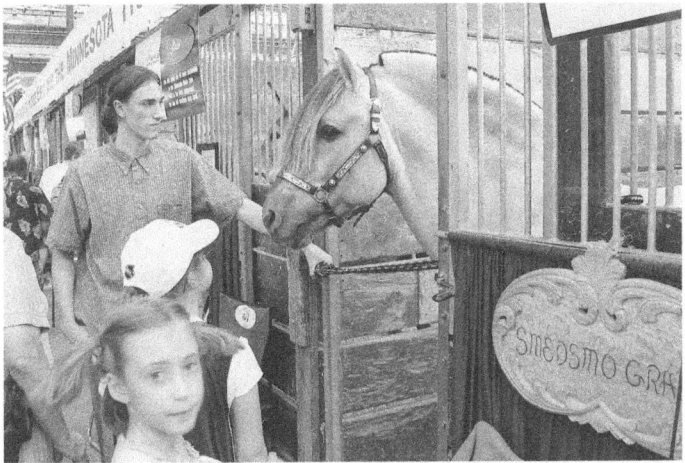

ABOVE *Stallion Smedsmo Gråen at the Minnesota State Fair.* Photo: ELSE BIGTON

I often walked by the aisles probably ignoring some beautiful horses in my search for a Fjord, but when I caught a glimpse of an upright mane, black and white forelock, and huge inquisitive eyes, I was pulled in as though by a huge magnet.

About five years ago, when I knew I would get a Fjord, I belatedly discovered a horse exhibition area tucked away behind trees at a small fall fair. The last event of the day was just ending and two Fjords were in the ring. I managed to engage the riders briefly and rub the face of one of the horses, but the riders (not surprisingly) treated me like anyone on the street. By then, I already felt so much a part of the Fjord community that their dismissal hurt, as silly as that was, especially for a fiftysomething adult working on her PhD. This book has a Fjord bias; I admit it. There are several reasons for my special attention to Fjords:

1. Fjords are often positioned as a good breed for a first horse because of their patient, inquisitive, and sometimes mischievous temperaments, as well as other characteristics.
2. It is what I know. Most of the learning I have done about horses in recent years has been about Fjords. However, much of the information in the book will apply to other breeds.
3. My Fjord is a great choice for me as my first horse.
4. Fjords are relatively short: typically around 14 hands.
5. Fjords are versatile, so if you start off thinking you want to be involved with Western sports, then realize you have become very interested in driving, your Fjord can probably learn both and a lot more.
6. I have spoken to many mature female horse owners with far more expertise than I have who have owned other breeds and are delighted to finally have a Fjord.
7. They attract attention. People are interested in them, even

if they don't know the breed. This can help you meet people and tap into communities of horse owners.

8. This is a rare and little-known breed that I feel deserves more attention.

THEME	SAMPLE TERMS
Calm	Calm, sensible, steady, quiet, stout, gentle, easy-going, even temperament, temperament beyond compare, mellow, Labrador-like, laid-back, patient, docile, warm, co-operative, freak-out resistant, nice personality, quiet, tolerant, friendly, kind, placid, safe.
Physical	Short: easier to tack up and mount. Strong, sturdy enough for heavier riders or those working on balance. Healthy. Athletic. VERY attractive. Just plain cute.
Versatile	Versatile: trail, dressage, jump, drive. Competitive at low-level dressage, eventing and driving. They do well in competitive trail riding. They foxhunt.
Attitude	Forgiving, curious, people-centric, very forgiving of our faults, easy to train.
Intelligence	Smart, rational animal, thinking horse, very curious.
Misc.	"Grandchildren love them!" "They love to drive as well as ride, so as you age, you can decide to drive rather than ride (less painful!). They can carry or pull as much as any large horse so you can take your non-horsey friends along in the cart!" "Cost: less in the long run than a 'free horse'" "I personally am not quick on my feet anymore. When I was younger I could dodge hooves or do much faster corrections. Now, I just want to be able to relax with a sensible horse, not that I'm lazy, just want to have fun with one, instead of constantly having to be alert all the time like I have to be with my half-Arab. Fjords suit me just right."

Table 1: Fjord Owners' Perspectives on the Breed

Fjords are a breed to seriously consider because they are small, versatile, curious, and people-oriented. Most well-bred and well-trained Fjords are extremely reliable. More than forty women who own Fjords (and other breeds) shared insights with me about the suitability of the breed for mature women. Several spoke about the risks of generalizing about any breed and the importance of training. If an individual horse is difficult, poorly trained, or poorly disciplined, their strengths become their detriments.

Table 1 shows the most common patterns in comments and stories about Fjords as a potentially good breed for mature women. The themes at the top were most common and those at the end of the list were only mentioned by a few women.

When you realize how many times some of these glowing terms were repeated, it makes the Fjord sound too good to be true. But it is important to hear some of the extra context these women shared, even though they wrote such qualifiers as "I am a true Fjord fan, so don't get me wrong."

The Caveats:

Pay attention to these valuable insights from experienced horsewomen with Fjords and other types of horses. I have tried to keep the spirit of their statements as well as the content.

- Horses are a risky business to enjoy in your old age.
- Be ready for work, and horses can hurt you, without meaning to of course.
- Some of the heavy Fjords stretch your hip joints like the Chinese splits.
- I do feel you have to have some horse experience in order

to be able to handle them well. My less experienced friends don't cope well with Fjords at times!

- A poor horseperson can have problems with any horse, and Fjords are quick to learn the wrong things.
- A Fjord is a good choice [for mature women considering their first horse] IF the horse is already well trained and prepared. Otherwise, with the strength of the breed, you could be in for some unpleasant surprises.
- Fjords are very, very smart and a newbie could get in a lot of trouble with a Fjord or any horse without some solid advice and mentoring.
- There are differences between a breed and a horse; all horses are individuals. I have had five Fjords and probably only two of them would be suitable for someone older without a lot of experience with horses.
- The Fjord breed is inclined to include more of the "right" individual horses, but although I love and respect the breed, no one breed is perfect for everyone, especially for beginners. Overall, the breed is inclined to be steady and kind (if trained properly and ridden often enough). But there are Thorough-breds that are good for beginners.
- Avoid "projects."
- Buy for current needs, not necessarily for an imagined future.
- A beginner might have a bit of difficulty finding tack to properly fit a Fjord.
- Have seasoned horse owners/trainers to get started.

In addition to these cautions, I heard stories that spoke to the character of Fjords and the ways in which people are pulled into relationships with these horses. One woman shared that without any previous experience, she and her husband trained their two Fjords in nine months to ride and to drive as singles and as a team. As a beginner myself, I am so impressed with the speed of those accomplishments.

Kathleen was browsing the Internet in her Florida home and was drawn to a picture of a horse at a pregnant mare urine (PMU) farm in Canada. PMU farms breed mares to harvest their urine and extract estrogen for pharmaceutical use. The PMU industry has been accused of mistreating horses and producing unwanted foals. Kathleen put the picture on the fridge so that she could enjoy seeing this Fjord mare. She had always imagined living in her dream home, sitting at a computer, and looking out the window to see her horses grazing in a pasture. Until she eventually explored the possibility of adoption and undertook the three-thousand-mile trip, she didn't realize that her dream would come true. She now blogs about life with Fjords, dogs, and family (not necessarily in that order) at cassidyapril.com.

And I like the way Pat summed up why mature women might choose Fjords: "Their brains! They are like a mature woman in a lot of ways. They have ideas and are pretty sure they're right. They're steady, strong and good-hearted."

I would like to wrap up this section with yet another reminder about how much there is to learn. In a recent conversation online, one woman spoke about how—in her view—Morgans and Fjords were not as solid and calm as they were many years ago. She thought increased interest in competitions, such as combined driving events (CDES) and dressage, were making the horses slimmer and hotter over time. Amidst the many comments were two from experienced breeders that caught my attention. I knew that in breed evaluations, conformation—the quality of body shape, bone structure, and musculature—was scored. Perhaps you have seen ads that say something like "Excellent, classic conformation evaluated as 81." And I knew that Europeans are very serious about which stallions are good enough for breeding. What I didn't realize was all the potential areas that can be evaluated and that different countries choose to focus on different things. So, for example, European Fjord evaluations include temperament, whereas North American ones do not. Lori Albrough of Bluebird Lane Fjords in Ontario described stallion testing in Europe:

> One comment really got my attention, when one poster said that they would gladly trade two blue evaluated Fjord horses for a pokey Fjord of yesteryear. This comment made me want to point out the difference in evaluation systems between countries.
>
> The North American system doesn't have a way to evaluate temperament or disposition. The conformation/ movement portion is essentially 10–15 minutes in-hand on the triangle, and the performance tests are presenting a 15-minute test mounted or driven by the horse's own owner/trainer/handler. This gives, in my opinion, limited opportunity for the judges to truly know the "inside" of the horse.
>
> Contrast this to the 30-day stallion test in Europe, where young stallions are brought to the station and left there for the 30-day duration, where they are handled daily by trainers they don't know, who are scoring these horses on EVERYTHING. This includes the horses' behaviour in the stall, manners, willingness to work, respect, cooperation with people, ability to learn.
>
> The young stallions in the station test are taught their basics in riding, driving, and draft work; they do

free jumping, riding outside in wide open spaces as well as traffic; they do basic dressage. Every facet of this work and how they deal with it is scored by their trainers. Even the vet gives a score for what the horse is like to handle!

Another Fjord horseman, Phil Odden, reminded me that all horses are good horses until you ask them to do something! He also pointed out that all evaluation programs have strengths and weaknesses, so each individual needs to bring their own knowledge and experience to the table to make informed decisions.

When you are considering a first horse, the way a breed is evaluated in different countries might seem way down the priority list of things to learn. But there are so many layers to learning, and unlikely topics might become very interesting or important in the future. By the time I bought a Fjord, I knew I was getting much more than a horse. I had a sense of how Norwegians feel about Fjords as an important part of their history and identity. I knew each Fjord had at least some of the strengths of that history: willingness to partner with humans, power, calmness, curiosity, intelligence, versatility, and perhaps a touch of mischief. Many breeds come with an equally rich history and with communities of owners who take pride in playing small parts in the evolution of that history.

Most women who shared their ideas in this section have Fjords they purchased from owners and breeders. But Kathleen chose to get a horse that might have gone to auction, perhaps to be sold for meat. This book does not go into depth about horse rescue. However, there are good reasons to rescue, and reputable organizations can help with the adoption process. In this section, I briefly deal with the benefits, risks, and approaches to successful adoption.

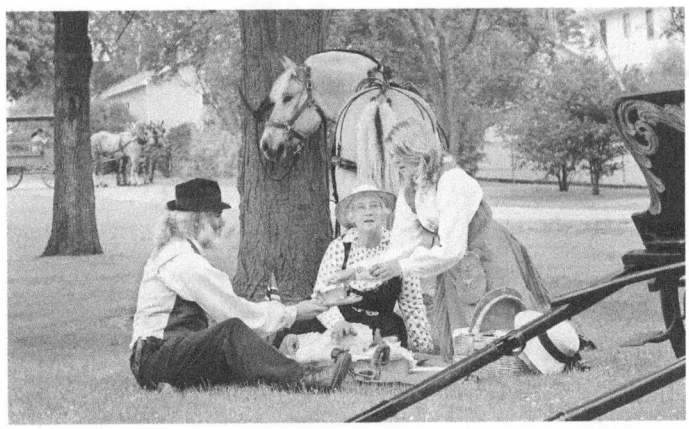

ABOVE A traditional picnic with a Fjord, a hand-carved Norwegian cart, and people wearing bunads (Norwegian costumes). Fjords are sometimes considered living folk art. Photo: ELSE BIGTON

To Buy or to "Rescue"?

So you have a preference for breed category and perhaps for breed. Should you search with the intent of buying a horse (from a current owner/trainer/breeder) or with the intent of adopting from a rescue centre? To begin with, use the terms "rescue" and "adopt" thoughtfully. Show respect for the people engaged in the difficult rescue work. They are the ones witnessing tragic situations, going to slaughterhouses, and working with the SPCA and other animal protection agencies. They deal with malnutrition, parasites, injuries, and emotionally wounded horses. They have probably poured countless hours into care before most of us might show up onsite and see a horse we might consider adopting.

The horses can be grouped into three overlapping categories: 1) horses that have outlived their purposes, whether that is racing, breeding, or being part of a farm that shuts down; 2) abused or neglected horses who have made their way to rescue organizations; or 3) horses in meat pens or slaughterhouses.

If you search on the web using terms such as "horse rescue organizations," you will find at least two types of listings. Some will include lists of organizations in broad geographic areas such as the United States and/or Canada. Other links will take you to specific sites from which you can adopt horses. I approached twenty such organizations to learn more about their day-to-day issues. I learned about interesting patterns in the people interested in adoption, the horses they want to adopt, and what happens after adoption:

1. The People: Most potential rescue centre horse adopters are mature women, drawn to the idea of saving a horse from mistreatment or death. Christine Hajek of Gentle Giants Draft Horse Rescue was one of several horse rescue professionals who told me about the importance of preparation. She said that most mature women who consider adoption "honestly have a romantic notion of saving some flowing-maned beauty and having this wonderful and love-filled connection. Few are prepared for owning any horse, let alone a rescue horse." Some of the women have totally unrealistic expectations. Rescue organizations receive requests such as, "I want a 6 year old dead broke horse of [insert special preferred rare breed and/or choice colour] and it has to be trained English and Western, safe for children, safe in traffic and on highways, it must be healthy and sound, and under $800." It takes masterful tact, patience, and a good deal of luck to move such people towards informed adoption decisions.

2. The Horses: Rescue horses often come with baggage, and the baggage might not be immediately obvious. Horses have superb memories, and rescue horses probably have unpleasant or fearful memories of humans. As reported by NBC news, Jill Starr, president and founder of Lifesavers Wild Horse Rescue, says that "horses can be very forgiving, but they never forget." Bad memories can be very specific: you may not hit the panic button until you wear a dark Stetson or pick up a crop or go into an arena for the first time.

Oddly enough, such "baggage" doesn't seem to be at the forefront of adopters' minds. Many are drawn to certain physical horse characteristics. These include showy colours, interesting markings, "romantic" or Baroque breeds, and young horses not trained to ride. A University of Kentucky study by Jill Stowe sheds light on the most adoptable horses. She looked at characteristics of adopted off-track Thoroughbreds and found that horses with fewer activity restrictions, that were sound enough to do some jumping, and that were young had faster adoption rates. She also found that grey horses were adopted about thirty-three days sooner than bays, and chestnuts twenty-four days sooner than bays.

3. What Happens After Adoption? We don't always know, but some rescue organizations require by contract that the horses be returned to them if the adoptive owners no longer want them. One rescue organization manager shared that despite putting a lot of effort into good, well-educated matches, the average adoption is in fact temporary—only three to five years in duration. She wrote: "I always try to get to the bottom of why a horse is returned and the honest answer is normally loss of interest, or the horse has now become aged and limited. So, most adopters are not really as altruistic as they wish to view themselves." Stowe's study found that, paradoxically, horses with fewer activity restrictions were more likely to be returned, as were greys. These findings suggest adopters give more weight to predetermined or aesthetic criteria than to deeper evidence of fit.

If you think you might like to go the adoption route, seriously consider the following pieces of advice from rescue organizations. As a matter of fact, most of these suggestions provide great food for thought, even if you buy rather than adopt:

▸ Do you really want to adopt, or would it be better for you to help rescue organizations in other ways, such as donating money, feed, or supplies? Horse sponsorship? Fundraising? Volunteering? All are needed.
▸ To learn about horse adoption, volunteer at a working rescue or horse farm to gain hands-on experience for at least six months before making your decision.
▸ Take riding lessons for six months to a year at a farm where you have to catch, groom, tack, and ride different horses. Learn about basics of horse care, handling, and training.
▸ Ensure you have the resources you need (see chapter 4), with extra emphasis on access to good coaching and training.
▸ Watch lots of training videos from reputable trainers. Some videos are free online or from a library; some can be purchased on DVD. You may be able to observe live clinics in your area.

When you think about the resources you need for work with your rescued or adopted horse, keep horse forums and other social media in mind. Horse forum members often post to let others know when a good horse is in a "kill pen" waiting for slaughter. And they also share when they have taken

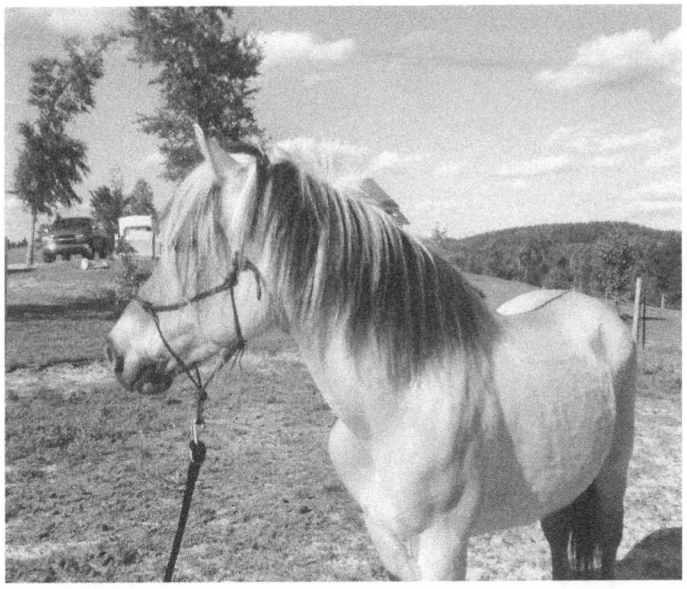

ABOVE Lars' stable mate had died of starvation before he was rescued.
People with the skills and resourcefulness to get horses like Lars back in shape
deserve a lot of credit. Photo: ELLEN BARRY

on a rescue horse, as did Ellen Barry. Ellen found a Fjord for
sale on Craigslist. The owner had owned two; one had died
of starvation and the other was very thin. Ellen brought the
horse to her property and posted pictures. She got him registered in the U.S. Norwegian Fjord Horse Registry and shared
his name: Lars. The owner of the horse's sister surfaced and
shared information about her horse's similar appearance
(including handsome zebra stripes on the legs) and temperament. Almost daily, updates appeared about medical tests
and procedures, successes, setbacks, and evidence of previous issues in this horse's life that surfaced in various ways. As
a hint of all the things you would learn as a horse owner, here

is a small segment of one update, this one relating to a visit
to the vet:

> His physical was OK. Too skinny but we knew that one.
> Conformationally correct, nice topline, nice big cannon
> bones, good feet etc. Vet was very happy with him. He's
> supposed to be dewormed again in 10 days for the last
> time. After that, just fecal egg counts and only deworm
> when necessary. He had a good sheath cleaning. His
> teeth were floated; no wolf-teeth present. He was tested
> for Lyme's; results in 3-4 days. Coggins done: results in
> a week. He got his Fluvac-EWT, his Pinnacle I.N., Flu-
> vac EHV4/1 and his West Nile Vax. He behaved like a
> good boy. Very docile, very cooperative. Trailered like
> a charm.

The amount of work involved with rehabilitating Lars
was obvious, with so many details, like "I have taken close
to ninety ticks off him. Thank God we have close to forty
Guinea fowl. Not a tick will survive them." And Ellen's disturbing report that both Lars's canines were shattered: "The
dentist couldn't even guess at that one." Ellen embellished
many of her posts with signature block "reactions" to this
new visitor from her other Fjords, such as: "Sam: HIS TAIL
IS NOT NICER THAN MINE," and "Kari: Oh, he's so gor-
geous. Does he see me?" After a big investment of effort by
Ellen, her vet, and many others, Lars was ready for a long-
term home: he is now the beloved trail horse of a family in
Tennessee. The new owners love Lars so much that they
bought a second Fjord.

To me, the story of Lars exemplifies the amount of skill
and commitment it takes to work with a promising but

damaged horse and how a forum can provide you with knowledgeable and supportive company during the journey.

Age and Sex

I asked people in forums about getting a mare versus a gelding. What did I need to know for this decision? People advised me that this was very low on the list of factors to consider. The right horse might be either. There are differences worth learning about, but I wouldn't factor them into purchase decisions unless you want to breed a mare.

Horses of different breeds seem to mature at different rates, or perhaps they are pushed into certain roles at different rates. A two-year-old Thoroughbred might be racing on the track, whereas a Fjord of the same age is two years away from being ridden. A Thoroughbred might be a retired trail-riding horse at seventeen, whereas a Fjord is going strong at twenty-five.

I wanted a Fjord with several years of training, so I wasn't looking for one younger than eight or nine. Perhaps the "right horse" for me would have ended up being much older. We might have retired from riding in tandem and been friends with all our feet on the ground after that. There is no single right answer, but make an informed decision for you.

Geographic Location

I have heard women say things like "Well, this was the best local horse I could find," or "I couldn't look at that horse because I'd have to travel." Would we say that about purchasing a vacation property or a boat or helping to find a college for a niece? Probably not. In chapter 5, you will read about different ways to cast the net widely and perhaps find the right horse some distance away. You may not have to do this.

Perhaps you want a Morgan, and the farm with the best reputation for breeding and training calm, reliable Morgans is an
hour away. This may work perfectly for you, but we aren't all
so lucky.

When I look back to my searching days, I found this to
be a real quandary. Fjords are rare, I was unlikely to find the
right horse nearby, I didn't have a lot of money, and I didn't
want to drain what I had saved over the years on airfare. And
I thought even if I were wealthy, how much good would it
do for me to fly around the continent with my rudimentary
knowledge and skills, where owners eager to sell for whatever reasons might convince me their horse was the right
one. Over time, I learned about many ways to search at a distance with a number of safety nets to help me find the right
horse without travelling.

POINTS TO PONDER

▶ Use your life experience to make wise decisions.

▶ Shop *seriously* for the right horse. How much effort would you put
into buying a car that you expect to have for a few years? At least
triple that.

▶ Learn more about groups of breeds, individual breeds, and generalizations about their characteristics, realizing they are generalizations.

▶ If you feel a strong emotional pull towards horse ownership, shop
strategically. Spend time with horses you *cannot* buy (at a riding stable, for example) and learn by talking to people and reading.

▶ Start to think about your horse preferences in relation to who you
really are and want to be at this stage of your life.

▶ Narrow your search, thinking about breeds, size, temperament, versatility, and so on.

▶ Think about purchase versus adoption, and remember it doesn't have to be one or the other. You can help rescue organizations in many ways.

▸ Even if you have horse experience, be extremely cautious about buying a horse that needs work. Leave that to the twenty- or thirtysomethings.

▸ Follow some of the rescue professionals' advice, regardless of where you might get the right horse.

▸ Don't let geographic distance limit your selection more than it should.

QUESTION TO CONSIDER

▸ Do you want to work with other people's horses for a few years, get a beginner's horse of your own for a few years, or get your "forever" horse soon?

"Some people talk to animals.
Not many listen though.
That's the problem."

A.A. MILNE

4 | Do You Really Have What It Takes?

DO YOU HAVE a Community?

For me, a learning community was essential. It doesn't seem to be critical for everyone, but think about this seriously. You will have so many questions and decisions, and if you learn on your own or from books, which are static, you are apt to make unnecessary mistakes. Also, social learning can be a lot of fun.

What do I mean by community? I am referring to a loosely defined group of people who interact with each other in order to learn about and improve their skill set in a specific topic, such as horse ownership. In workplaces, we might use the term "community of practice." This term grew out of research at the Institute for Research on Learning by Étienne Wenger, who had been brought in as an artificial intelligence expert, and anthropologist Jean Lave. Their collaborations led to new ways of thinking about learning while doing with others—or "situated" learning—in order to improve.

Communities are fluid; they evolve. Some people will be active and central; some may watch from the edges. Leadership will emerge in various ways.

What takes place in communities? Here are activities I have experienced or heard about. Hundreds of approaches to learning are possible. A group:

1. chooses a training video series (much like a book club). They gather monthly to watch a video and to show progress they have made with some of their horses over the past month;
2. creates an online space, such as a Yahoo or LinkedIn group, where members can post questions and others can respond and react, regardless of where they live;
3. holds a retreat once a year to gather on a ranch, have fun, and ride trails;
4. arranges for a coach to teach once a week (I'd put this sort of learning on the essential list);
5. sets up horse games in someone's ring for a light-hearted competition;
6. sets up a test day with a judge to practise the skills one would use in a show and to get feedback on strengths and areas for improvement;
7. arranges a workshop with an expert invited to instruct people in some skill (such as equine massage or hoof trimming or monitoring saddle fit); or
8. books motel rooms for a big trade fair with presenters and clinicians, where attendees can go to sessions during the days and compare notes each evening.

You may be able to join in these sorts of activities before you become a horse owner. The learning will help you weigh options and plan for the type of horse you might buy.

Do You Have the Resources?

There are many types of resources to consider, including money, time, energy, maturity, and external resources such as facilities and services. The following lists of resources may seem daunting. But if you are reading this book, you probably have many of these items in place or have the capability and capacity to build your resources over time. Your horse will appreciate the confidence you develop in the process.

Financial Resources: The following list is not all-inclusive but can help you decide whether you can afford a horse. Women who are passionate about horse ownership often find themselves stretching their resources, regardless of how much income or savings they have. This list is based on the assumption that you will not have income or tax deductions—such as coaching or running a bed, bale, and breakfast—associated with your horse ownership. It does not include the original purchase and transport costs.

Hay can be a major expense. If a horse eats about six to twenty-five pounds per day (the lower figure would be combined with pasture) and bales are $5 to $20 each, the cost per year will range from $200 to $3,400. The variation in hay cost estimates comes from many factors, including geographic location, type of hay, when the hay was cut, and other issues such as drought. The weight of "typical" square bales can vary by more than twenty pounds. Some horses may have pasture for part of the year, some may have no access to pasture, and some should not have much or any grass. The costs in this chapter probably capture typical expenditures but may not reflect your area or needs.

The contents and costs of pellet or extruded feed, sometimes referred to as "grain," vary. This is worth some research, as there can be risks to feeding your horse too much or too little. These feeds are carefully prepared with different levels of protein, fat, selenium, and other nutrients. You often have to do a bit of arithmetic. One bag may look similar to another and be less expensive. But by the time you figure out how much your horse weighs, how many pounds they recommend for a nine-hundred-pound horse, and how many cups of pellets make up that weight, you might only use a cup and a half a day from the expensive bag and eight to ten cups from the other. Talk to feed store nutritionists, salespeople, and local horse owners to begin learning about options. And follow up with your veterinarian to see whether she/he agrees with your plans.

Farrier costs vary as well. Some people do their own trimming and save money. However, owners are rarely as skilled as a good farrier or barefoot trimmer, and amateur trims can cause serious problems. Some owners keep their horses barefoot all the time (as I do). Some have the farrier hot-shoe the front feet only; some have all four done. Farriers may charge more for horses requiring special shoes. If your horse develops hoof problems, your costs will go up—hopefully temporarily—and may even involve trailering to a specialist until the issues are resolved. Estimate spending $200 to $1,700 per year. Take very good care of your horse's feet.

Vet costs are unpredictable. Have your horse's teeth floated by a professional, which is a procedure to smooth the teeth with a file, and consider whether you want the vet to do vaccinations and worming. Learn basic first aid and signs of when a vet must be called. It is the emergency care that wreaks havoc with the budget. You can avoid surprise expenses by having insurance. Estimate spending $150 to $900 per year, regardless of which route you take.

Expenditures for tack vary even more widely. One person might spend $3,000 on each of two saddles and another might pay a fitter to adjust an old saddle in a friend's barn. Estimating tack costs is a bit like estimating how much a city girl will spend on shoes. Some people just can't get enough. I've never enjoyed shopping, but now I find I can't resist a tack and supplies store, where silly things like a gold-coloured fly mask tempt me.

Similarly, one person might buy dozens of extras for grooming, fly management, supplements, barn accessories, and more, whereas another gets a few basics and picks up other things second hand as they are needed. In addition to the well-known horse supply chains, check out independent dealers; consignment shops; second-hand sale fundraisers for 4H programs, therapy barns, and the like; and local swap days. Even if you are bargain-minded, expect to spend an average of $100 per year. U.S. Equestrian Federation members spend upwards of $7,200 annually on horse-related products. This figure comes from the Equestrian Channel, with a mission "to promote and support tomorrow's Olympic talent," so their expenditures will be higher than average.

Another cost consideration is that of a companion animal. Horses are herd animals and many argue they will not be happy as lone animals. There are people who successfully keep lone horses; some thrive and others cope. If there are horses on an adjacent property, or if you would board your horse where there are others around, this would not be an additional cost. However, many people buy or care for a companion, often an older horse but sometimes a donkey or goat. Some horses bond strongly with dogs as well.

And don't forget the costs associated with learning, coaching, and training. Coaching involves you and your horse learning together. I have lessons weekly when the weather is good enough for the coach to come over. It is common for owners to send their horses to trainers for periods of time, but my mare is well enough trained that I haven't had to spend money there. I have bought books, attended one clinic with her, audited others, and gone to horse expos to watch clinicians. I have seen women who really wanted to do some of these things but couldn't afford to. I am not wealthy, but I saved for a long time and spend very little on things such as clothing, restaurants, entertainment, and vacations.

Don't feel as though you need to get all the details worked out years in advance. Human resources consultant Sharen Howarth entered into horse ownership in her forties through lessons, leasing, and boarding. She found it very useful to create a budget for each step of the way.

Time and Energy: Are you willing and able to invest the required time? Or perhaps I should ask are you *driven* to invest the required time? A horse isn't a motorbike or set of skis that you get out of the garage periodically and hop on. If you aren't passionate about owning a horse, and the drive to the barn is a nuisance, and you don't work with your horse enough to get better or deepen the relationship, you probably shouldn't own a horse.

Your energy will ebb and flow to some degree. Figure out what dampens your spirit (being cut off from communities would be devastating for me). Figure out what motivates you. If you get stuck, work with that motivation. Call your friend, watch the great video, sit in the pasture and remember what drew you to the dream of horse ownership. Get a sports psychologist. Talk to a person who would do anything to have a horse. Do whatever it takes to replenish your energy.

Recently, I had been in a bit of a slump, I felt as though my relationship with Bocina wasn't quite right, and I couldn't figure out what to do. She and her companion, an older Thoroughbred mare, were in a small dirt and grass ring, and I was holding the Thoroughbred while her owner put hoof hardener on her feet. Like most Fjords, Bocina is very food-oriented and was mowing the green grass at her usual startling rate. As I worked to keep the Thoroughbred relaxed, I felt Bocina's head settle on my shoulder from behind. She just stood there quietly, occasionally gently nuzzling, until we finished treating her companion's hooves. This gesture reassured me that there are many, often-unexpected ways, of recharging your confidence or motivation.

Maturity: Maturity is a nebulous but important concept. Perhaps reflections on my *not* being ready for horse ownership will help:

As a teen, I was so sure I would own horses. But having been flat broke at various times in my life, I set aside dreams of buying a horse to develop a career, save for a home, and raise children. In the early 1980s, my husband and I and our two young children moved to a rustic acreage large enough for horses. Sometime around then, I learned of the Fjord breed. These were hardy, versatile horses that didn't require green Kentucky-like pastures with white fences. They were reputedly good horses for almost anything, including riding, driving, and logging. I pictured a Fjord in the forest when I looked out the window. Sometimes, I would be lucky enough to see one at a fall fair, and they took my breath away.

But I knew I was not yet financially or emotionally ready for horse ownership. Many years before, when I was working for a vet, a young woman came in with a perfectly healthy kitten to be euthanized because she was moving out of province for a job. The vet carried out the request without question. On that day, I swore I would never get an animal of any sort without being quite sure that I would be a responsible, kind, long-term "owner." So, I didn't get a horse in the 1980s; we moved back to a city where I could find work and I pushed the dream into the back of my mind.

Unfortunately, as I wrote this book, I heard dozens of stories about women who make spur-of-the-moment decisions (interesting horseback riding roots in that metaphor!) without gaining the maturity needed for wise decisions. Here is one of the tamer stories: "Just last night, a new horse arrived at the barn. A handsome, 'sweet and nice' quarter gelding. And who is the owner? A woman in her 50's. How many lessons has she had? Three total. Where did she find this horse? In a field." Statistically, their relationship doesn't have much chance of lasting.

I have always had a passion for learning, which is so important for horse ownership. Since the 1980s, I have also become more patient, resilient, and adaptable—all attributes that have served me well.

Drawing loosely from the emotional intelligence literature, think about your strengths and areas for improvement in the following:

1. Are you reasonably self-aware? Do you notice when emotions are sneaking up on you? Do you know your strengths (and have you checked those perceptions with others)? Are you able to tap into your state of mind and energy level and ensure that your "inside" is coherent with your "outside"? (Horses pick up on this.)
2. Do you behave responsibly? If you are dealing with negative emotions, do you swim twenty laps or stack hay bales,

or do you bury the emotions or let them simmer? Do you believe in your ability to work through challenges and overcome them?

3. Do you tap into your environment? Read body language well? Are you empathetic? When you watch social dynamics, do you have a sense of how people's (or horses') interests, needs, and power dynamics are at play?

4. How well do you work with others? Do you enjoy meeting people? Learning about them? Discovering common interests and building deeper communication? If someone were to snap at you for borrowing a lead rope, how would you react?

If you have any big issues in these areas, you probably know it. If you aren't sure, ask some friends who are likely to be honest with you. It would be a good idea to work on problem areas before you get a horse. That isn't to say that the learning and growth will be complete when you do get a horse—they are masterful teachers in all these areas if you are open to the ongoing growth.

External Resources: We have explored the idea of community (where you live and online), and later in this chapter we talk about where to keep your horse. Some of the other things to consider include: services (a veterinarian, farrier, coach, feed sales); facilities (shelter, food storage, ring, indoor ring, round pen); and opportunities (trail access, events). There are certain services, facilities, and opportunities you won't want to live without and others in the "nice to have" category. Take a close look at the items you consider critical. A good horse vet is likely to be one of those.

As you consider these very important elements, look not only at what is in your area but also at the depth and breadth of the expertise. With the veterinarian example, consider these two very different scenarios and note the potential benefits and red flags.

1. You live just outside a small city, within four hours of a veterinary college. There are many vets in the area, and three work with horses. Two have very good reputations; the other arrived recently and is less of a known entity. You are in an area of small acreages where many of your neighbours have horses.
2. You live in an isolated area. As a matter of fact, let's put you on an island where you have to trailer your horse on a ferry for forty-five minutes as the first step to travelling anywhere. There is a vet on the island with some horse experience, but she mostly works with small animals. Two other people on the island have horses.

Think carefully about the implications of these two rather extreme scenarios. You don't need to be near a veterinary college, but you are lucky if you are and you will find some things are simpler and/or better when there are good services nearby.

My situation is closer to the second scenario than the first. I live on an island, though not as isolated as the hypothetical island above. I made sure there was a good vet, and he works primarily with large animals. He seems to be well settled into island life and gets lots of business. He is fine with people combining requests, so he might see two horses on one property and charge one travel fee, for example.

Isolation comes with both drawbacks and stimuli for people to work together. A recent horse injury illustrates this. A friend was caring for a horse while the owners were away, and the horse broke through a weak part of a fence and ended up injuring herself badly. The vet was away, but another woman who is a paramedic stepped in. They did some first aid work, got the horse in a trailer, and the paramedic (with her valuable community connections) had the ferry held so that they could get to the emergency veterinary hospital as quickly as possible. They did all the right things quickly and successfully.

Before I moved to the island, I also checked to be sure there was a certified coach to help me learn with my new horse. I corresponded with a generous, talented young woman with an honours degree, an organic garden where she saved and planted heritage seeds, a job as an editor as well as a coach, work experience in Canada and Europe (and I could go on). If it hadn't been for her, I don't think I would have made the move. She died suddenly at the age of twenty-two about a year and a half after I moved to the island. She remains an inspiration to me, and I often think of things she taught me. Environments are not static. You can plan perfectly, but you cannot predict perfectly.

Are You Developing a More Informed Plan for Purchase?

You have been reading and talking with friends and former strangers who have helped you weigh options. You are narrowing the search. Your early list of preferences (and I encourage you to make one) might look something like the one in Table 2.

This kind of planning helps you ask good questions. The questions don't have to be polished. I recall one online community post where a woman asked something like "I have just discovered Fjords and in all the pictures, they seem to be either eating or kissing their owners. Are they really like that?" A great discussion ensued.

ITEM	PREFERENCE	COMMENTS
Type	Warmblood	Not too big
Breed	?	Versatile
Mare or Gelding	?	Important?
Age	6-15	How old is old?
Cost	?	
Amount of training	High	
Types of training	English	Learn more
And so on…		

Table 2: Purchasing Decision Checklist

Location, Location, Location

Where will you keep your horse? At the risk of oversimplifying, there are three options: 1) your own acreage, 2) self-board and 3) full-board. Most people in Canada keep their horses on their own properties. In some countries and in most urban centres, people board their horses elsewhere. "Self-board" and "full-board" describe the two ends of the spectrum for boarding options. There are variations; the specifics below describe the extremes.

If your horse is on your own property, you can gradually decide what facilities you want to develop. In many cases, there will be shared private, community, or commercial facilities nearby (such as a riding ring) that you can use. Basically, you will need to store and provide feed and water, manage manure, and provide shelter.

When you self-board, you take care of your horse on someone else's property. You buy the food and bedding and do your own feeding, grooming, farrier booking, vet booking, worming, manure picking, and so on. There will probably be other horses on the property, and you might work out some arrangement for sharing chores.

With full-board, the owners or managers of the facility care for your horse. Food and bedding are included. Your horse is fed three or four times per day. If your horse is in a stall overnight, the stall will be cleaned, and he will be turned out and brought in by staff. Your horse may be blanketed as needed. There might be extras included, such as one riding lesson per week for you. You will have access to facilities such as indoor and outdoor rings, a round pen, and a wash rack.

Sometimes, your horses will be "amused" by your decisions. Before I got Bocina, I offered to volunteer at a Fjord farm to learn more about caring for horses on your own land. Unfortunately, they had just closed their farm and only had their stallion with his new miniature donkey companion animal on site. But I visited anyway and learned a lot. The farm's owner, Errol, described ways in which his Fjords had taught him about facilities. The pattern was the simpler the better. He kept "downgrading" facilities based on what they liked best. Their preferred shelter ended up being a windbreak made by lumber nailed to trees. Despite stock tanks and bathtubs full of water, they preferred to drink from a shallow stream that ran across the surface of the ground for much of the year. Similarly, I have a friend who built a very nice run-in shed for her miniature horse. She is not a carpenter, and this was a Big Deal. The mini is afraid of the shed, runs in to grab mouthfuls of hay, and goes under the porch when it rains.

When boarding, if you are lucky enough to have several options, you will have to make many decisions. Costs can vary from almost nothing to several hundred dollars per month. I consider the criteria listed below to be essential, regardless of where you are on the boarding spectrum:

▸ Reputation: Are the owners or managers trustworthy, ethical, reliable, and "compatible?"
▸ Health and Safety: Does the facility seem free of any problems that could affect your horse's health/safety, or yours?

What do I mean by "compatible"? The people with whom you would interact need not be the warmest or friendliest people you have met. You need not want to invite them for dinner. They might be no-nonsense, efficient managers who seem a bit distant. They should have good references. You want to have a good sense that they care about you and your horse and know what they are doing, and that you can interact with them comfortably.

The following list includes additional considerations for choosing a boarding facility:

▸ Affordable
▸ Resident manager onsite
▸ Appropriate shelter
▸ Space for horse to get some exercise
▸ Appropriate level of access to grass
▸ Appropriate, individualized feeding
▸ Easy watering provisions for cold weather
▸ Tack room (temperature controlled, rodent proof)
▸ Outdoor ring
▸ Indoor ring (Olympic-sized if competitive)
▸ Round pen
▸ Equipment (jumps, barrels, as needed)
▸ Coach(es) and/or trainer(s)

- Access to trails and/or hacking area
- Good veterinarian and farrier
- Wash stall/racks/bay (with warm water)
- Hot walkers
- Washrooms
- Electricity
- Viewing area for lessons; coffee machine
- Lockers

Details for items in the list above will vary depending on your interests and needs, your climate and your horse. For example, one horse might thrive on several hours of grazing; another would be healthier with no grass or less than an hour of grazing per day.

If you are working up to having your horse on your current or future property, boarding can be very educational. I had no idea how useful rings and round pens were when I first got my horse, and I hadn't realized how wonderful a covered ring or arena would be in the long, wet winters where I live. I can't imagine ever owning such facilities but would recommend someone in this climate be within riding or trailering distance from them.

Manure management deserves mention. This may seem like an odd topic to consider before getting a horse, but it is important for many reasons.

1. Many books about property set-up focus primarily on facilities, so many novices are slow to learn about the issues involved in manure management.
2. If you have not spent much time around horses, you will be amazed by the vast quantities of manure they produce.
3. Poor manure management can make enemies of neighbours or even limit your ability to keep the horse on your property.

4. Poor manure management can have serious environmental impacts. Just as many businesses are starting to think beyond profit to social and environmental well-being, horse owners need to consider their influence on communities and natural environments.
5. Even if you are boarding, you may have responsibilities or options for input regarding manure management.

The Langley Environmental Partners Society has documented issues arising from poor manure management, including:

- Unsafe drinking water because of ground water pollution or well contamination
- Animal health problems such as the spread of disease among livestock
- Increased numbers of insect pests
- Destruction of aquatic habitat vital to the survival of aquatic life
- Difficulties with neighbours because of the smell and unsightliness of manure
- The loss of the right to farm in a rapidly urbanizing area

Manure should be piled away from streams or other water, covered, and properly composted to make "black gold" for growing superb flowers and organic vegetables as soon as possible. If you will be keeping your horse on your property, think ahead to how you will handle manure in ways that avoid social conflicts and environmental impacts. Fortunately, manure is in high demand by gardeners and farmers. Near urban areas you might be able to sell manure, and in the country people might pick it up from piles or even in the fields. But you need to take the lead to create and maintain your strategy. Don't plan to have a horse on your property if you cannot manage manure properly.

POINTS TO PONDER

- ▶ Reach out to potential communities (face to face or online) to get a sense of the support available to you, by approaching local horse owners, coaches or vets, or asking questions online.
- ▶ Make a list of the strengths and resources you already have.
- ▶ Draft a list of "must-haves" for facilities.
- ▶ Document any potential gaps in resources.
- ▶ Make a plan for where to keep your horse and consider what pros and cons you envision with that arrangement.
- ▶ Make a plan for effective manure management.

QUESTION TO CONSIDER

- ▶ What concerns you the most about your ability to get and care for a horse? Can you think of three people or groups who could help you work through those concerns?

*"What we find changes
who we become."*

PETER MORVILLE

5 | Narrowing Your Search for the Perfect Match

YOU UNDERSTAND the resources you will need; you think you are ready for the commitment; you have decided where you would keep a horse; and you have a better idea what sort of a horse you want. You are no longer satisfied by riding your friend's horse or taking lessons on school horses. You think a purchase makes more sense for you than adoption. You are ready to start shopping!

This chapter has two sections, one that deals with searching in person and the other that addresses searching online. Shopping for a horse is strangely similar to the human dating scene (apparently). Everyone used to meet each other in person. Everyone used to get their horse from the nice farmer down the street or the famous Thoroughbred breeder with whom they corresponded by mail. Now, for better or worse, most new couples first connect via the Internet, for reasons ranging from busy schedules to the fact that common interests may have nothing to do with geography. If a neighbour were to ask me today about Fjords for sale, I don't think there are any I would recommend for viewing within a daytrip from home (although I did know of one a few months ago who is enjoying his new local home). However, I usually know of some potentially good options I have found online.

If you are reading this chapter, you are probably an Internet user. But some of you might be relative beginners and others quite advanced. If you're a novice, recruit a friend or relative or neighbour's son or daughter or anyone who could sit with you and help get you started. Or if you are a do-it-yourself learner, you might try a beginners' site such as the Senior's Guide to Computers (seniorsguidetocomputers. com).

Searching in Person

In her *Fjordhorse Handbook*, Carol Rivoire provides a checklist of things to observe and do when shopping for a horse in person. She provides details about the following tips:

1. Visit the breeder's farm unannounced at a time when the barn chores would be complete. Look for signs of good (or poor) management.
2. Check out the quality of pastures and fencing.
3. Look at the condition and demeanour of the horses.
4. Ask to see one or more horses handled.
5. Ask about veterinary and farrier records.
6. Look to see whether the manes have been cut. (Fjord specific.)
7. Ask about the horses' bloodlines; the breeders should know these well.
8. Pay attention to what the breeder tells you about each horse and to how they speak about each individual.

Collectively, these tactics should give you a sense of the quality of the breeder's/owner's farm. This quality can influence the health and temperaments of horses in many ways.

When you go to see a horse, pay attention to what you *don't* do, or aren't encouraged to do, when you visit. Long-term horse owner Mary Ofjord shared several stories about red flags she didn't spot in her less-experienced days. Such as the time she went to see Buck, and when they "drove over to the farm and he was already hitched and in harness (red flag #1! unseen by us)." Later, during the inspection, when they asked whether Buck had been ridden, the owner put an old saddle over his back, left him in the driving harness, left the blinkers on, and let Mary's husband sit on him. How many red flags there? They didn't know enough not to buy Buck, and although it all worked out, there was a lot of drama en route to relative safety and pleasure. If there are things you want to do with the horse, try them, or at least have the current owner demonstrate them. Don't fall into the trap of thinking you are a nuisance: "Oh, they already put the bridle on; it must have been easy; I don't want to make them take it off again." Even when you take lessons, you are normally expected to catch the horse, groom the horse, put the tack on the horse, and so on. If you want to buy a horse, you want to see the owner handle the horse and you also want to check out how the horse behaves with everything from coming in from the field to having his feet cleaned.

Although I have never encountered this personally, I have heard stories of sellers being very deceitful, to the point of doing things like drugging a high-strung horse. As sad as I am to say this, do not automatically trust someone you don't know or wasn't recommended by reputable sources.

Another fabulous tip from horse owners is to take a friend or relative with you. Ideally, this person will know *you* as well as horses. One of my friends almost bought a gelding she really liked, but her husband said, "Don't you think you will want a horse with more zip than that?" He was right. She chose another horse, and she still got to enjoy the gelding because he was a great choice for one of her neighbours. Again, it saddens me to say this, but I have heard of poor advice from seemingly objective advisors. There is an expression in the U.K. horse trade: "There's a drink in it for you." Some of those "drinks" can be very pricey when dealing with expensive horses. But even a trainer might encourage you to buy a horse, knowing some training and thus income for them will come along with that decision. We all like to think everyone is open and honest, but I have also heard stories of people who are open and honest and are then marginalized by colleagues. Revealing unethical practices can be a bit like blowing the whistle on Wall Street.

Searching on the Internet

Good Internet access and research can be hugely helpful in expanding and then narrowing your list. There are two key types of resources on the Internet: 1) "static" websites such as farm websites that do not allow for comments and conversation and 2) more dynamic or social sites such as forums, bulletin boards, and social media. The static sites are like a book or newspaper article. They push information out, such as descriptions of breeds and ads showing horses for sale. The more social sites are more like a luncheon. They allow you to comment, ask questions, and help others. I have used Fjord examples to illustrate the resources below.

Websites

Through website searches, you can expect to find horses for sale with locations, descriptions, and prices. In some cases, you will be able to filter the lists according to criteria such as breed or location. You will see many listings that are not right for you, but you will learn in the process.

What does each ad talk about? Not talk about? Years ago, I listened to a gardening show where the guest spoke about what is not listed in seed catalogues. For example, a tomato variety might be described as having perfectly shaped, bright red fruits, but the catalogue doesn't mention flavour. Does the horse ad read "simple to catch" but neglect to mention behaviour under saddle? Does it say "has been ridden and driven" but nothing about how recently, how often, or with what sorts of training? Keep in mind that omissions may have as much to do with the skills of the people writing the ads as the qualities of the horse.

With your critical thinking hat on, explore some sites. For example, do a Google search for "Fjord horses for sale." The first link that came up for me was Equine Now (equinenow. com/fjord.htm). On that site, click on location and choose "California" from the drop-down list, which includes any or all U.S. states and Canadian provinces. The number of listings will change; when I did that search there were nine results: six sold and three not yet sold. In the Equine Now search site, you can sort and filter in many ways. For example, shift the breed to Morgan, restrict the list to geldings, and sort by size.

There are many other similar websites, including:

HorseClicks(horseclicks.com)

Horsetopia (horsetopia.com)

Dream Horse (dreamhorse.com)

Some websites simply list farms and ranches, which may have horses for sale. And, of course, there are localized horse sites (in our area we have one called Island Horses) and more generic sites such as Craigslist and Kijiji (which may include livestock for sale).

What are the trends in prices? In doing searches for Fjords, I noted three patterns related to cost. Untrained horses were relatively inexpensive. Unregistered horses were usually less expensive. And—although a novice searcher might not notice this—many of the larger, well-known breeding farms where high-quality horses would probably be more expensive were rare or absent. The relationship between price and training appears to be similar across all breeds. I spent more on my mare than I originally anticipated. But by the time I found the perfect match, I knew I wanted a well-trained horse. I didn't have skills or experience as a trainer, nor did I have the kind of assertiveness and confidence a friend used to train her Fjord from scratch, even though she was a novice. Also, I knew if I got a well-trained horse, I would usually know that the mistakes were mine, rather than second-guessing where things were going wrong.

Think about the math. Fjords are often started under saddle when they are four, but they have been handled and have done groundwork, lunging, and the like for some time before that. Let's say you buy an eight-year-old horse who has been handled and trained on the following schedule: three hours per week until age four; five hours per week until age eight. If you account for the trainer's time at $20 per hour (very modest if you consider the years of training, practice, and paid coaching they have had), then that means more than $33,000 has been invested in the horse, not including capital investments in the farm, hay, supplements, vaccinations, hoof trims, bedding, barn help, and so on. So if that horse were for sale for $15,000, how would that value compare with the cute yearling filly being sold for $2,500? As a rough estimate including capital and operational costs, the eight-year-old has an investment of $81,000 (you are "saving" $66,000), and the filly has an investment of $9,100 (you are "saving" $6,600, and you have a lot of work ahead of you). What if you don't have the skills and resources to raise the filly? A beautiful young horse may be difficult to place, just because she got a poor start with training. Even more importantly, think about the cost of a gift horse, which can be the most expensive kind. I was told of a woman who said, "She was quiet when I rode her." Her belated advisor said "Yep, quiet, depressed, starved, wormy and ten months pregnant."

The relationship between price and registration probably varies more by breed. Learn more about what registration means for your preferred breeds. Fjords are one of the very pure breeds; cross-breeding is strongly discouraged and cross-bred Fjords cannot be registered. In their home continent of Europe, governments regulate which Fjord stallions can be used for breeding. There are ways of classifying the best horses. When a horse is registered, you can visit the registration site to learn about the quality of the horse's ancestors. Even with horse breeds such as the American Quarter Horse, which is an unapologetic blend of breeds, the quality of ancestry can be important for reasons ranging from performance to health to resale value. However, there are good unregistered horses, and in some cases unregistered horses can still be registered.

Why are many well-known breeders missing from Equine Now and similar websites? If you walk into a run-of-the-mill department store in your area, you expect to find useful products, but you don't expect to find top-of-the-line goods. If a top-quality manufacturer wanted to get rid of some stock, managers might find other outlets rather than be associated with lower-end products, or they might simply find it problematic to be selling higher-quality goods beside lower-quality ones, with no easy way to talk about the differences. When you get to know a breed, you will learn about reliable breeders and trainers. They tend to have their own websites and sell by reputation. There are undoubtedly some great horses on the big multi-breed sites, but there is *less assurance* of finding a great horse. So your skill level in selection becomes more important.

In addition to the large horse classified sites, you may stumble on farm sites that become focal points for horse sales. For the Fjord breed, Willows Edge Farm is one example. On their site, they say: "Even if we personally don't have the perfect Fjord horse for you, we know there's a Norwegian Fjord out there for you…that's why we offer for others to list their horses for sale below as well."

Forums and Social Media

If you have not worked much online and are not aware of online communities related to your horse interests, it could be helpful to connect with some tech-savvy friends or relatives for some mentoring. The more contextual your questions, the more helpful such groups can be. For example, let's say "Mary" has a question about saddle shopping. Here are three different ways she can go about it:

1. What saddles are for sale in my local area? *Websites will work fine.*
2. Is an Australian saddle good for trail riding? *An Australian saddle supplier website will be a good start.*
3. I have an English saddle for my Fjord and wonder if I should get another saddle for trail riding. A friend said Australian saddles are good. My horse has low withers and he varies in weight. I have a problematic knee and wonder if an Australian saddle feels much different than an English one? *This is a highly contextual question. In a good forum, people with expertise will ask lots of questions to learn more about Mary's plans for trail riding,*

her horse, the nature of her knee injury, and more, and will provide information about saddles with tentative recommendations.

Many well-established sites (such as Yahoo, Google, LinkedIn, and Facebook) have built-in forum-like tools. Technology is changing rapidly, so as you read this book, the group options may be different for you. Some forums may have been created by members using different software (such as WordPress or Ning) and might have better content for you than ones you find in the sites listed above. Your tech-savvy friend could help you search for existing groups. You could also call breeders or talk with people in tack stores and ask if they are aware of such groups. If you have to find good forums on your own, start by searching with keywords such as "forum Quarter Horse" or "horse listserv" or "horse forum Wyoming" or whatever interests you. Look around a bit to judge the quality of the conversations. Even as a novice, you will get a feel for the expertise of members and the quality of their contributions. If you are really passionate about learning and helping others to learn, it only takes modest technical skills to start a group and see whether it takes off.

Some large forums hold a huge amount of collective expertise. Members may be veterinarians, equine event judges, nutritionists, barn managers, and so on, and they dig into technical detail as needed. For example, during a recent two-week period, ECHorsekeeping Yahoo group members posted questions, answers, and references about equine ophthalmology, stabilized versus freshly ground flax, hay analysis, magnesium supplements, fly control, and several other topics.

If you are active with any social media, mention your horse interests so that other interested members can find you. Cindy Giovanetti is a horse owner in Texas who makes extensive use of Facebook for learning. Although she has owned horses through much of her life, she says she bought Oden—a 13.2-hand Fjord gelding—as her "old lady horse." "I had to either get something gentle or get out of horses," she told me, and she is very glad she did the former.

Cindy is training Oden and learning some new techniques herself. She posts videos on her site, and comments on what went well and where she had some problems. Others encourage her through comments or by "liking" her success stories. Often she gets tips about how to improve her technique. Other comments focus on learning; she appreciated the comment: "Some of your followers are your teachers and some are or will be your students."

The microblogging tool Twitter is another way to share information and connect with people who have similar interests. In my mini-biography on Twitter, I focus on my consulting work, but I also mention I own a Fjord horse. (Because of space restrictions, my bio text used to read "Fjord owner," but several people were in awe of my owning a body of water on another continent.)

This allows other users to search for "horse" and have the option of contacting people like me, as Bobbie Sale did recently. Bobbie and I have since had several valuable conversations, exchanged pictures of our Fjords, and even found out they were related.

I recently looked back in my email horse folder for examples of how communities had helped me to learn. I was literally wide-eyed; I had forgotten how many questions I had asked and how many people had responded. I do vividly recall the sense of community and how welcomed I felt with my beginner questions. Almost always I got a range of opinions in response, but I valued that hugely. It was a great way to learn—and was often funny as well. Pat Holland wrote my favourite response to a question I asked about companion animals. At the time, I thought I would have Bocina on my small rural property and was considering a miniature donkey as her companion. Pat said:

> I'm going to stick my neck out—and say from past experiences you may NOT even need a companion. Yes horses are pack animals, etc. I have had good experiences with the care of singular horses and ponies. It can be done, and they will not die, and they thrive.
>
> I have found when one seems to think they NEED a companion for their horse it often leads to a major domino effect.
>
> You buy a buddy for the one horse, then the pecking order rules come into effect. One horse is assertive over the other, so then you feel sorry for the horse getting picked on. So you get him/her a companion because horse #1 is beating up companion #2. Now we have three: a REAL herd is made. Two become best friends, and the 3rd is an outsider, thus a 4th animal is brought into the mix. Then one is a mare and babies are soooo cute, and Mr. Smith down the road has that beautiful stallion... hummm baby on the way. Eventually you have 16 horses, a new barn, indoor, trainer, trailer, tack room full of stuff, farrier and vet bills, and a husband that says: "didn't we only buy one?"
>
> OK I tend to elaborate, but I will add that I once had a client who did indeed purchase a mini donkey for companionship for their Fjord. Every time it rained, the donkey would stand at the gate and bay, bawl or whatever they do, until I brought HIM in alone to a stall cause he didn't like to be wet! No joke.
>
> Good luck.

I mentioned earlier that there are several quality-control techniques to help you search for your horse at a distance. I have recommended using search engines to become familiar with what is out there, watching for registration and the quality of breeding in a registration listing, determining trainer reputation, and building and using communities as sounding boards. There is another tip that was invaluable for me. Through forums, I learned about people with great reputations as matchmakers—they were especially skilled at linking a purchaser with the right horse. I contacted one of them when I was close to making a decision. Without charging me, she watched videos, did a bit of research, and provided feedback, offering to do more work for a fee if I needed it. She was confirming my intuitive choice, which was extremely reassuring. We lived thousands of miles apart, but when we corresponded, it was like having her visit in my kitchen.

If you find good forums, like the Fjord horse lists are for me, treasure them and help them thrive.

POINTS TO PONDER

- There are at least two ways to shop for a horse: in person and online.
- Do everything you can to find honest, reputable farms, breeders, and sellers.
- Get ongoing advice from knowledgeable friends and colleagues or horse professionals.
- You can think of the costs of buying a horse simply as short term, or also as long term. Good choices up front can minimize costs ranging from training to veterinary care.
- The Internet can be very helpful. And you *can* feel as though you like, respect, and know people on forums, even if you never meet in person.

- Consider using social media to build your network.
- As you get close to making a decision, try to find the good "matchmakers."
- Treasure your communities; care for them like you care for your favourite garden plants.

QUESTION TO CONSIDER

- What is your personal reaction to looking for and learning about horses using the Internet? Why do you think you have that reaction? How might it help or hinder you in your learning?

*"Shopping is really complicated
if you are a girl."*

HELEN SALTER

6 | Getting Other Essentials in Place

YOU HAVE DECIDED. You are getting a horse. You have a place for your horse on your own property, or you know there are boarding options, or you are ready to negotiate an agreement whereby a current owner would keep your horse temporarily while you complete preparations. What else do you need to do to prepare for the big arrival?

History

Learn, document, and file as much as you can about your horse, including information from the vet check if that is being done at a distance. Not only will you have your own questions, you may get unexpected questions from your vet, coach, trainer, friends, and family. Some facts are obviously more important than others: veterinary records trump his favourite treats.

When I got Bocina, I received an electronic (scanned) record of veterinary and related care for the previous few years. I transferred this information into a Word file so that I could update it easily. It included:

- vaccination history with diseases and dates in a table,
- deworming history with products and dates in a table,
- dental procedures (all were floats) with dates and vets' initials, and
- farrier procedures (all were hoof trims) with dates and farrier initials.

Know exactly what your horse has been eating and when. I added a nutritional section to the document described above, in part so that I could compare previous supplement composition with brands available on the West Coast.

I also know about her ancestry through the breed registry, which is important for various purposes, including choosing an appropriate stallion if I ever breed her and perhaps for health history if problems ever arise.

Know about the saddle and other tack. What bit is your horse used to? Does he like it? Is there a saddle that fits well? (This is particularly important for breeds that are difficult to fit, such as Fjords.) What sorts of tack has he experienced? Has he been ridden Western? English? Has he been driven? Get some more detail on these things. Statements like "He's very skilled; he did competitive barrel racing for years" could flag that there may be physical issues now or in the future.

What training has he had and how recently? How did he do? If he "used to" do a lot of something, did he stop because he didn't like it, or was he injured, or did he reach a high level for his breed and the owner didn't want to push?

Some history may be unavailable, especially for rescue horses. Probe to reveal the mysteries, such as: "He doesn't seem to like going into a ring; we don't know why," or even more subtly, "He seems to be best on trails." What does "doesn't seem to like" look like?

Transport

If you are very fortunate, you may lead your horse down the road. Perhaps you have a trailer already and can look after a short trip yourself. I often see community members ask for help when moving a horse across the country. Someone might be delivering a horse to one part of the country and pick up another for the return trip.

Like many people, I needed to arrange for commercial transportation. I did some research on the web and by contacting haulers. In the long run, I was more comfortable with the recommendation from my horse's previous owner, based on lots of personal experience. Interestingly, the preferred hauler was not easy to find through regular advertising channels. Depending on the starting point and destination, you may be hiring more than one hauler. They seem to know other haulers and partner with specific haulers they respect. So if someone is recommended, but they don't come to your part of the country, talk with them anyway.

When horses are hauled short distances, they usually stand in one place (as they would in a typical privately owned trailer) with cross ties on their halters, so they move very little. For a longer trip, they usually go into a box stall, where they are not tied to the wall. Horses use a lot of muscle balancing in a trailer, and for a long haul, a box stall is far more comfortable than a standing stall and worth the extra money (remember to have enough resources to be proud of yourself as a horse owner). The hauler will ask you about the size of your horse, as some haulers have different sizes of standing and box stalls.

Insurance

There are companies that provide insurance for horse injuries, illnesses, or surgeries as well as for tack and for rider injuries. My mare was insured when I bought her, and I have carried on with the insurance. I surveyed about fifty horse owners and got close to fifty opinions. One of the most specific recommendations was to get enough insurance to cover an episode of colic and to ensure you have a credit card with a substantial available limit. Predictably, some respondents had spent thousands on insurance and never used it (I am one of those); some did not have insurance and had dealt with expensive emergencies. As one woman summed it up succinctly, "It's a crap shoot." The key factors to consider when deciding whether to purchase insurance are:

1. The type and age of the horse. Some breeds are perceived to be lower risk for medical problems. Also, a thirty-year-old is more likely to encounter health issues than a fifteen-year-old. That said, most insurance companies will not cover older horses.
2. Uses. Showing, competition, and riding in areas with risks (such as heavy traffic) are indicators that insurance is particularly important.
3. The financial value of the horse. People with a $20,000 (or $200,000) horse seem more inclined to purchase insurance than people who bought their horse for much less.
4. Your attitude. Would you be sad but bounce back easily if a horse were euthanized because of a serious, expensive but treatable injury? Or would you be devastated by having to make that choice?
5. Your knowledge and experience. I got insurance partly because I didn't know what I didn't know.

6. Your financial situation. Some people would need to drain all their savings and much more if they were faced with a $10,000 vet bill. Others could manage the expense without hardship.

When you research insurance, be sure you understand the procedures when there is an incident. They may say "call us right away," but what exactly does that mean? If you have a horse in agony, do you have to wait for their approval before treatment or euthanization? If you forget to call for a few days, is the insurance valid? If you have insurance, post the details with the company's contact information and basic procedures so that anyone can find them. I have this information on my fridge and on the wall of the tack room where my mare is boarded.

Food

Sometimes you want to know what a previous owner did because you want to make a change. Last year at a fall fair, I saw a very obese Fjord who was so heavy that I hung around hoping I could learn more and perhaps make a respectful suggestion or two. Through some eavesdropping, I learned that the owner was relatively new and was well aware of the health risks. She had managed to get about 250 pounds off this gelding, who was perhaps 14 hands tall. The previous owner simply hadn't understood that different breeds have different needs and had the gelding out on full pasture with his other horses. I congratulated her on her efforts and told her how glad I was she'd taken on this gentle guy who had a wonderful personality and deserved a great home.

If your horse was well treated by his previous owner and is healthy, try to match his feed types and feeding schedules as closely as possible. I say "as closely" for several reasons. Perhaps your schedule only allows two feedings per day and your horse is used to four? I recommend you invest in a few of the nets, bags, or homemade devices that slow the consumption of hay. These have many benefits, including:

1. Slow consumption of hay mimics natural grazing behaviour and is better for digestion and health, especially for horses who gain weight easily;
2. Most horses seem to enjoy the challenge, and it gives them something to do for a longer period of time than gulping a pile of hay;
3. You make fewer trips to the barn or field if you have no other reason to be there;
4. Much less hay (if any) is wasted;
5. Nets can be used in many locations: attached to a wall, hung from a tree, hung in a trailer, and some can be put on the ground; I sometimes relocate mine for a sort of scavenger hunt; and
6. For people who want or need to soak hay for their horses, nets can easily be immersed in a container of water and then hung to drain.

I initially bought two Nibblenets by mail order, because I had read in Fjord horse communities that Fjords are very tough on slow feeding products and these stand up well. I bought one with 2-inch openings and one with 1.5-inch openings, not knowing whether she could eat properly from the smaller mesh size. I put two heavy-duty eye screws into the shed wall and all her hay went into the Nibblenet. I later learned she could probably get hay from 0.25-inch openings, if they made such a thing! Find out whether your horse is used to particular slow feeding products, including grazing muzzles.

Once your horse is moved, you will almost inevitably buy hay from a different farmer than your horse was used to. You could either compare hay tests before your horse arrives, or learn more over time about any important differences. If you don't have hay tests, do your best to match the hay using less scientific criteria. For example, if you know your horse was thriving on first-cut orchard grass, try to find that in your area. If you cannot, go for another type of grass, but stay with first cut (which means the first harvest of the year from a hayfield). Whenever possible, make a transition gradually. And do not make a huge shift, such as switching from first-cut grass to third-cut alfalfa-grass mix. There is always more to learn about nutrition, and many feed supply stores have a nutritionist on staff.

The brands of supplements your horse is used to might not be available in your area. Bocina's usual pellet feed was not sold in my location. I got the ingredients list to determine exactly how much protein and minerals were in the previous mix, went on the web, and talked to feed store staff to find the closest equivalent.

Finally, be sure you are set up with lots of fresh water and salt on demand.

Tack and Equipment

This could be a whole book (and, of course, there are many books out there with good information about tack). Below, I list the essentials I had when Bocina arrived. In chapter 8, I describe items that were critical or especially helpful for me during that big initial learning curve with groundwork and English riding.

The main components for basic riding are: saddle, bridle, and crop or dressage whip. Much to my surprise at the time, my "right horse" was a dressage horse. I didn't realize basic levels of dressage are more like taking your horse to the gym than preparing to compete in a specialized sport. So to learn to speak her "training language," I needed a dressage saddle, bridle, and whip. Of course, I had bought a "beginner's kit," from the Greenhawk chain, which included a crop and not a whip, but that has been useful, too.

Saddles

A saddle fitter once told my friend Dan Maxwell that a saddle "is the only piece of sport equipment shared between two athletes." It deserves very careful attention. If you are new to saddle shopping, be aware that saddles are made to fit both horses and riders. If you have ever worn a pair of shoes that fit poorly on a long walk, you get a small sense of what a horse has to endure with a saddle that does not fit. This is extra sad when you realize that horses—as prey animals— hate to show when they are in pain.

Ruth Hanks, who is a manager with a saddlery, talked to me about the implications of getting older and often gaining some weight in the process. A heavier rider might need a nineteen-and-a-half-inch saddle, but she points out it would be cruel to put this saddle on a horse when the useable part of his back is only seventeen inches long.

A friend of mine got a great little hybrid Western trail saddle that had been custom made for someone she had never met. She copied the serial number and wrote to the saddle maker. Her note went something like this: "Tell me if I am correct. I have bought your saddle number ####. It was made for a woman who was about 5'2"–5'4" and weighed about

130–150 lbs. It was for a horse that had a broad, flat back, and was possibly a gaited breed." She was right on with every point. Not many of us can afford a saddle that is absolutely perfect for horse and rider, but you want to be as close as possible.

Some breeds, including Fjords, are notoriously difficult for saddle fitting. I had witnessed online discussions about treeless saddles, adjustable saddles, saddles designed for wide horses, and so on. There were disturbing posts about expensive almost new saddles being sold cheaply because they didn't fit. I wanted to be extremely careful with the saddle purchase. Eventually, Bocina's owner, Lori, told me she had a Schleese saddle for sale because it was a bit too long for Bocina's stablemate. It fit Bocina well and could be adjusted there by a saddle fitter for a perfect fit. As Lori and I were a similar size, I thought the saddle would probably fit me reasonably well.

To me, it was hugely valuable to have a professional fitter work with someone who knew the horse better than anyone else. It pushed me into a higher price bracket than I envisioned, but I had seen so many people struggle for months to get a really good, safe fit. I highly recommend a similar approach if you are a relative beginner, especially if you live in an isolated area. If you aren't so fortunate, try to work with a company or individual that will lend you a saddle, and have qualified people help you determine whether it fits well.

A magical product I encountered was the waterproof saddle cover. I use it when there is a bit of drizzle or the threat of rain. This protects the leather saddle very well. Some people have synthetic saddles, which they use all the time, for rainy days or for swimming with their horses. There are other accessories available for rider comfort, too, such as sheepskin or gel pads.

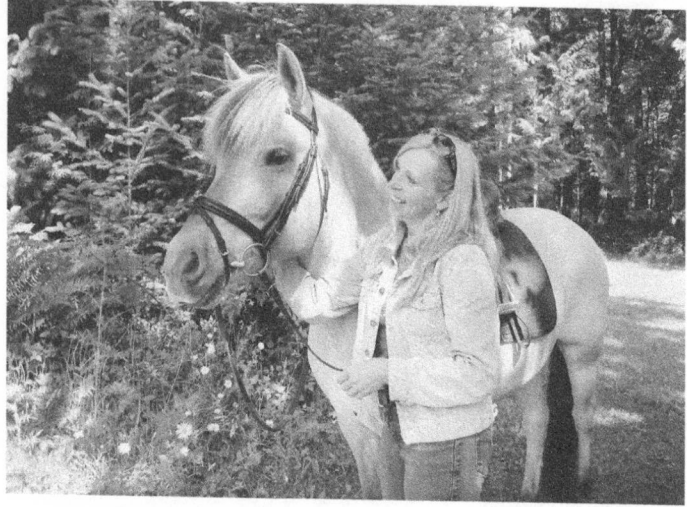

ABOVE Bridle with a mild French link snaffle bit, customized for the short but solid Fjord head. Photo: ALICE MACGILLIVRAY

Bridles and Bits

These may not be as difficult as a saddle purchase, but a good fit, comfort, and effectiveness are important. I used an approach much like my saddle purchase. Bocina wears a full-sized bridle with shortened cheek straps, as the Fjord breed has a short but solid head. Her bridle fit her perfectly, and Lori said Bocina loved the bit. However, her bridle was not for sale. Brubacher's is a Mennonite harness and tack shop within driving distance of Bocina's old barn (they sell online as well). Mr. Brubacher borrowed her bridle and quickly replicated it.

The saddle and bridle purchases might seem extravagant, as I spent at least five times what I thought I might, yet I think of them as two of the best decisions I made. Most importantly, they helped to ensure the comfort of my horse. These decisions also helped to focus my learning curve. With every decision I made to minimize unnecessary changes for my mare, I greatly increased the likelihood that successes and setbacks had to do with *my* skills, behaviours, or attitudes. If she didn't respond to an aid, for example, I wasn't worried about whether it had to do with a new bit or uncomfortable saddle pressure.

Dressage Whips

I am still not used to the term "whip," as a dressage whip is typically used in a gentle way. I carry one when I ride, because it is a handy supplement to leg aids (using your legs to give directions to your horse). A dressage whip is similar to a riding crop but longer. At first, I did not realize how different pieces of tack fit together. I know much more now, but I made early mistakes, such as buying a standard-sized saddle pad, which would have been fine with an all-purpose saddle (or "no-purpose saddle" as a friend calls them) but would not work with Bocina's dressage saddle and obviously would not have worked with a Western saddle. A dressage saddle covers more of the side of the horse than an all-purpose saddle, for example, so you need a larger saddle pad and a whip longer than a crop to easily touch the side of the horse.

Basic Groundwork

The main components for basic groundwork are: halter, rope, and gloves. Many horse people believe it is very important to work with your horse on the ground as well as under saddle. The simplest reason for this is that your horse needs to respect people on the ground. The farrier and vet come on foot; you groom your horse on foot, put on blankets and tack, and lead her from field to field. Some horses figure out that they are much stronger than humans, and perhaps their human backs down. These horses become dangerous quickly. Another reason for doing groundwork is because it is a way of checking responsiveness. Will your horse move forward and back, disengage the hind end, move her shoulders over and carry out other useful moves based on your body position, touch, or energy? All these behaviours are important under saddle, and groundwork can be a short warm-up before a ride.

Halter: There are many styles of halter, made with leather, nylon, or rope. I stayed with the leather halter Bocina wore at her previous home. Everything I read recommended never leaving a horse in a field with a halter, so I removed it after working with her, despite the fact that she sometimes lived with horses who wore halters in the field.

Rope: Lori steered me to a thick, soft cotton rope, and I love it. It feels good, and may be safer than a synthetic rope if a horse pulls away quickly.

Gloves: You can't have enough. I started with three pairs, and the ones I still have are stretchy, durable cloth on the back with leather on the palms. The leather is great protection against the reins and the rope and a nice texture for giving Bocina a rub.

Lunging Equipment: I did not get any lunging equipment right away and am still learning a lot about how to lunge a horse properly.

Horse Blankets and Sheets
When Bocina came west, she had been shaved completely, so she didn't get too sweaty when working (this is called a full-body clip), and she was going to be trailered through some very cold weather. I have driven through Rogers Pass, a high

mountain pass through the Rockies, on many occasions without being nervous, even though there are frequent snow and avalanche hazards. But I must have pictured her going through the pass more than a dozen times, almost holding my breath as I did so!

For the trip, she wore a borrowed medium-weight stable blanket (a garment that covers the horse's chest, back, sides, and rump, and is designed for indoor use), and I bought a winter turnout (which looks similar but is waterproof and designed for outdoor use) for her when she arrived. The West Coast climate is much milder than Bocina's previous home, but because of her clip, I put a winter turnout on her almost every night through that first spring. I had purchased an Irish-made turnout, as I had heard that most manufacturers in drier climates just don't understand West Coast rain.

Riding Apparel

Helmets: In my view, helmets are essential. I had a very basic but good-fitting new helmet ready for Bocina's arrival. I know there are many photos of good riders without helmets, but I believe it is never worth the risk. Some of us remember professional athletes playing dangerous sports without wearing helmets. Now there is more awareness of the effects of concussions, especially if the injuries are not properly diagnosed or treated, or if someone sustains repeated concussions. There is a movement to replace the classic dressage hats in high-level competitions with helmets. Helmet use seems to be an especially sensitive issue with Western riders—there just isn't a history and culture of helmets. It doesn't matter if you are a great rider or riding the calmest horse in the world: wear a good-fitting helmet that has never suffered an impact. It could be a gift to yourself, the people who care about you, and your horse. My first coach on Gabriola Island, Kelly, was a great role model for this. Once while riding on a back road, we switched positions: I dismounted and she mounted. Then she realized she hadn't put on a helmet. She was visibly shocked and told me it was the very first time in her life she had forgotten. That stuck with me.

Boots and Half Chaps: I didn't mind buying used boots, because I generally tried to buy inexpensive things so that I could learn what I liked and then maybe move up to higher-end products over time. So I scoured consignment stores and found a lovely pair of used paddock boots. The price was great, partly because they were covered in mud, and partly because they were in the low-profile, low-demand boys' section. The boots had a full, attached leather tongue, and after a good scrub, they looked fabulous (temporarily).

By this time, I had a pair of half-chaps as part of my beginner's kit. Half-chaps slip on over your boots with an elastic strap across the base of your foot and zip up over your calves to protect your legs from stirrup strap friction. Half-chap sizing can be a shock. I hover around the boundary between healthy weight and overweight. My regular clothes are around size six to eight, or small to medium. However, my half-chaps are size *extra large*, and I cannot fit into many tall boots. If you've been out of the saddle for a few decades and no longer have calves like an eleven-year-old's, don't take the sizing personally.

Riding Clothes: These are important to keep you comfortable. Good clothes protect you from the weather, as well as from abrasions or blisters, and allow good freedom of motion. I started off with inexpensive riding pants or "breeches." Some Western folks think they look silly, but the grippy seats help you sit securely in the saddle, and the snug-fitting design allows you to feel a horse's subtle movements. Most Western riders wear jeans, but select jeans with certain characteristics such as no rough inside seams. I didn't buy any other specialty items of clothing, except for an inexpensive reflective equine safety vest for riding on roads. Be careful these vests don't rub against and scratch your saddle.

Grooming and Leather Care

This category may be the equivalent of shoes in a woman's wardrobe. Canadians alone said they spent about $100 million on horse grooming and care products over a one-year period. In *The Fjordhorse Handbook*, Carol Rivoire provides excellent detail about why and how to groom your horse and adds the caution: "Adults must be really vigilant regarding excessive shampooing if there are little girls on the farm, because there's nothing little girls enjoy more than shampooing a horse. I swear, they'd rather shampoo than ride."

I started with basic grooming and leather care materials, including:

- Rubber and plastic curry combs
- A body brush (I used the thick horsehair curling brush I had on hand)
- A hoof pick and brush
- Shampoo
- A detangling product for the tail
- Sponges and towels
- Scissors and clippers I already had on hand from my vet assistant and dog grooming days

If you have more than one horse, be sure each has her own brushes and hoof picks to prevent the spread of bacteria, fungal spores, and other problems.

Over time, I added to my supply as I learned more about what Bocina and I liked and needed. I did not buy one of the very stiff synthetic "dandy brushes," though I see them in tack boxes all the time. They just seemed too rough, and other tools seemed to do the job. I was relieved when I eventually read Allan Hamilton's view in *Zen Mind, Zen Horse* that they "are suitable only for scrubbing toilets."

I also bought good-quality saddle soap and a recommended leather conditioner for the saddle, bridle, and halter. I received conflicting advice about how often to use them. I decided to go with the recommendation to wipe down tack with a damp cloth after every ride, use saddle soap every ten rides or so, and apply leather conditioner about once per month.

Unless you are in a very isolated area, buy the minimal essentials to start with and expand gradually, based on what you like and what you learn.

POINTS TO PONDER

▸ As you prepare for your horse's arrival, focus more on health, safety, and function than on appearance.

▸ Get all available information about your horse, including veterinary records and diet and registration information.

▸ Decide whether to purchase insurance for death, injury, tack, and so on.

▸ Choose respected, knowledgeable people to move your horse.

▸ Find experienced advisors to help you adapt the ideas in this chapter to your situation.

▸ Plan to minimize changes to your horse's diet.

▸ Get basic equipment and tack in place; go for quality on items important to health, safety and comfort that you know will fit; be economical with other items to see what you like and need.

QUESTION TO CONSIDER

► Have you started a journal? List items where you do not want to compromise quality, even from the start. How will you make wise investments for those key items?

"'What day is it?'
'It's today,' squeaked Piglet.
'My favorite day,' said Pooh."

A.A. MILNE

7 | The Big Arrival

YOU'VE BEEN WATCHING the driveway and pacing for some time, and finally a big trailer pulls into the property. You have the stall or run-in shed ready. There is hay in a net to ensure she could nibble on hay over a long period, water in a stock tank, and wood shavings on the floor. The hauler opens the trailer door and a thousand pounds of energy steps out, taking in every tiny detail of the unfamiliar surroundings. What next? You are standing at the transition point where dream becomes reality.

Enlist Experienced Help Right Away

Have an experienced horse person there for your horse's arrival. Have a coach lined up to support you at your level, whatever that might be. Have your vet out to check your horse, especially if you have the horse on trial subject to a vet check done at your barn. Have a stack of horse books on your bedside table. Do whatever you can to remind yourself you have lots of support.

The Horse You Buy May Not Be the Horse You Get

When I bought my mare, she had a wonderful structured life. She did some trail riding and showing but was typically ridden five times a week in an arena on her home property and was expected to respond to an excellent rider's aids promptly and appropriately. She got ten to sixteen pounds of hay each day, depending on pasture, served in four feedings. Her afternoons were spent in big open fields with other Fjord mares. She was groomed well each morning. Her stall looked like it was from *Better Barns and Gardens*.

She was also very gentle—so gentle that she always ended up on the bottom of the pecking order among the other horses, even when a new filly arrived. I rode her in the

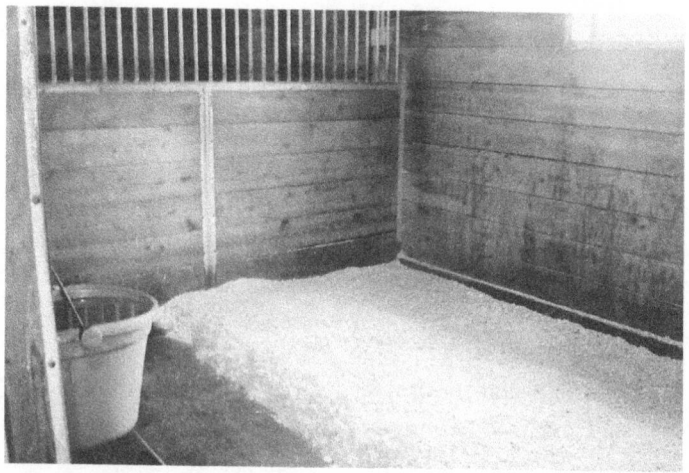

ABOVE *A typically beautiful daily stall-cleaning job by Brandi Kingsmill at Bluebird Lane Fjords.* Photo: ALICE MACGILLIVRAY

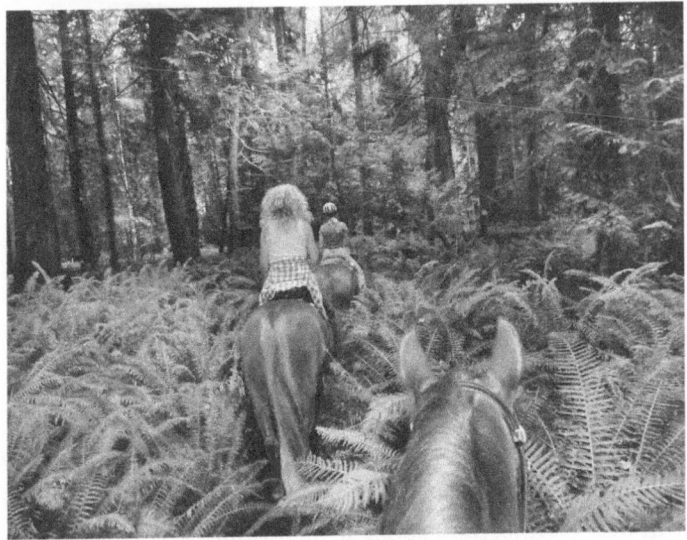

ABOVE *A backcountry trail ride through sword ferns on Canada's west coast.*
Photo: ANNE MABBERLEY (*on Jack*)

arena, and she behaved wonderfully, filling in the blanks as needed: "Maybe she means a leg-yield? I'll try that."

Then she arrived in the lush, temperate rainforest of Canada's west coast. The dense conifer forest must have seemed so foreign after her Ontario and Pennsylvania homes in big open fields with deciduous trees.

Bocina quickly concluded that "Thar Be Dragons on the West Coast." They lurk by narrow trails and in forests and they hide in roadside litter, cattle, donkeys, and even chickens. To make matters worse, her new rider apparently didn't know what she was doing (so true). I was fortunate she didn't bolt during our early trail walks (I led her at this stage and climbed in the saddle later). I didn't even know to carry a crop or whip when we went out for walks. When

I could feel her body tense with fear, her head high and her eyes darting around in the woods, I would speak to her softly and reassure her. When she started to walk too quickly or jig, I would ask her to halt and praise her when she did. If it felt like things were getting well beyond my skill level, I would try to make it plain it was my decision to turn around and walk back as calmly as possible. On the narrow trail, she often invaded my space, and I didn't deal with that very effectively, but there were no mishaps. Given the width of the trail, perhaps I should have walked her behind me, but that would have come with some risks as well. Perhaps I should have stayed on the driveways at first, where there was room for each of us to have our personal spaces. Regardless of what tactics you use, be—and look—as confident as you can. You may be uncertain about several things, but be sure you understand where some of your confidence lies. Take something like protection of your personal space and insist your horse understands that boundary. Do this with kindness and with uncompromising firmness. By showing your horse her boundaries, you help her to relax.

When I started to ride Bocina, I had to hold up her head and neck for the first year: if I did not know exactly how to ask for longitudinal suppleness (an important shift in her body position that I describe in chapter 10), she was not going to give it. Her essence was still there: she was mischievous, tolerant, curious, patient, and responsive when she had a good rider on her back. She was kind—once, when I mounted and she walked away (which she should not have done), I lost my balance and almost fell off. She stopped, lifted her head, and braced her neck so that I was able to retrieve my balance.

As we went through these experiences, I realized the human-horse-environment system had changed, and we were immersed in that change. She wasn't quite the same horse I had bought, and I wasn't quite the same person who had bought her.

How did I deal with this? In part 2, I outline some of the things I learned.

POINTS TO PONDER

- ► Have experienced help in place for when your horse arrives.
- ► Feed your horse frequently to make sure he will be able to keep his digestive tract active. Choose products such as nets to slow the consumption of hay, for example. This can help to prevent ulcers and other problems.
- ► Make the new surroundings as trustworthy and familiar as possible.
- ► Be as confident as possible. You don't have to know everything to make firm, informed decisions.

QUESTION TO CONSIDER

- ► How will you become comfortable with the unpredictability of people, horses and environments all influencing and changing each other?

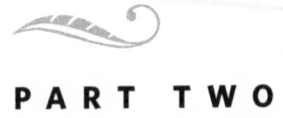

PART TWO

The Awakening
The
Relationship
Begins

YOU WALK OUT towards the pasture on a sunny Saturday morning. Your horse lifts his head and watches you approach. He trots towards you. You know he has eaten; he isn't coming for food. He is coming to meet you. You ask him to step back from the gate and he does so willingly, making a soft, throaty nicker as you come into the field. You invite him into your space and he pushes his warm muzzle against your chest and hand. Then he gives you a look like "So, what are we going to do?!?" This is quite unlike your entry into the pasture the day before, when he looked up briefly, kept grazing, and gave you a go-away gesture with his ears and neck when you stroked his side. What's different today?

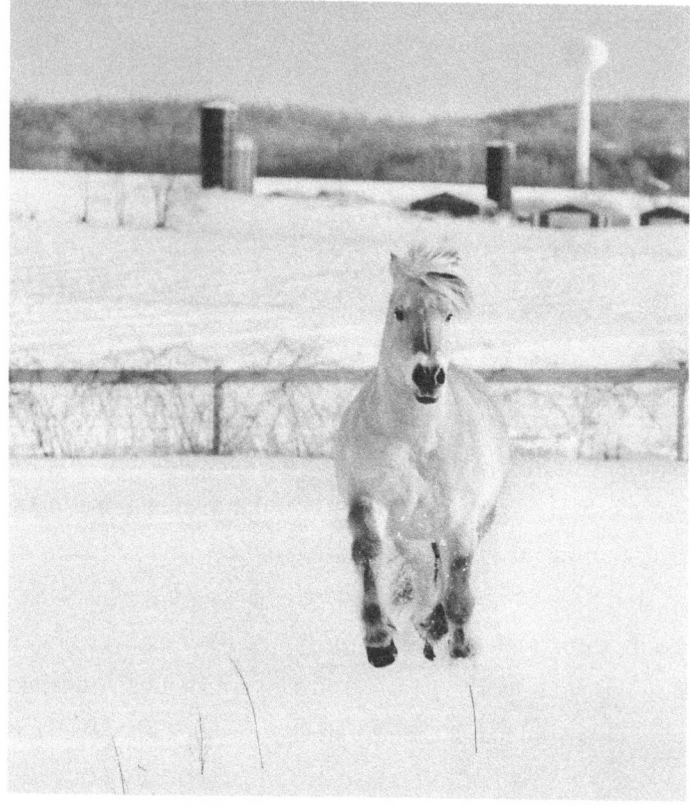

Your horse coming to greet you can be a powerful experience. This is Bocina's magnificent sire, Prisco, nicknamed Dutch. Photo: P. SPEAR

Such is the day-to-day reality of horse ownership, especially during that learning curve when we aren't as adept as we would like to be at understanding our equine companions. Building a relationship isn't like choosing a brand of turnout or deciding whether to buy first- or second-cut hay. This is much more nuanced work.

You may have heard the old adage that changing a tire is much simpler than changing a career. It is relatively simple to provide steps for increasing the likelihood of finding a horse that will be a good match for you. Guiding the development of a healthy relationship is not as straightforward. If it were, there would only be one or two guides for childrearing and another couple for marriage. And with childrearing and marriage, we are talking about relationships within a species. Human-horse relationships have different dynamics. Perhaps some of you are offended that I compare childrearing and horsemanship? I do not mean to imply they are equal. Quite the opposite: I want to emphasize that they both take considerable effort and each comes with some distinctive challenges and rewards. It is remarkable that literate, linear, logically trained, globally dominant predators can associate with—let alone become close with—big, fleet-footed, right-brained prey animals.

"And woman is the same as horses: two wills act in opposition inside her. With one will she wants to subject herself utterly. With the other she wants to bolt, and pitch her rider to perdition."

D.H. LAWRENCE

8 | Women and Horses

I WAS ABOUT FOURTEEN when I read *The Naked Ape*. I was fascinated by zoology and wanted to be a veterinarian. I thought Desmond Morris was brilliant. I loved the book, until I read: "The horse is a powerful, muscular and dominant animal... viewed objectively, the act of horse-riding consists of a long series of rhythmic movements with the legs wide apart and in close contact with the body of the animal. Its appeal for girls appears to result from the combination of its masculinity and the nature of the posture and actions performed."

I was furious (fourteen-year-old girls can do furious very well). I knew the relationship between women and horses was much more profound than that, but my understanding was intuitive. How could I build a logical argument to refute Morris? I filed the experience away in a don't-assume-scientists-are-right category, alongside the scientific assertion of the day that birds were colour blind, despite the fact that my budgie would only play with yellow pencils.

While reflecting on this chapter, an equine consumers' guide arrived in the mail. I think it's good to do the occasional bit of quantitative research, so I counted the number of photographs of men and women in the guide. Marketers often know their audiences well; this might be thought-provoking if not informative. Many pictures were so small that gender was ambiguous. I counted every person recognizable as male or female. In some cases, photographs were printed two or more times in different parts of the guide, in which case I included each duplicate image.

There were 95 images of men and 137 of women. In other words, it was a forty-sixty split, implying the publication is of more interest to women. More intriguing were the ways in which the men and women were portrayed in ads, or what they were doing in real life as horsemen or horsewomen. The characterizations below are mine; the people in the photographs might not have described themselves as I did.

Of the ninety-five people identifiable as male, there were:

· Thirty-six WWI soldiers (because of a special feature inspired by the film *War Horse*),

· Thirteen cowboys on the range or in Western competitive events.

That took care of more than half. The remaining men and boys were VIP observers at a competitive event, jockeys in races, competitive jumpers, trainers, stable owners, or in other professions such as veterinary medicine, mounted police work, horseshoeing, or fitting saddles. There were also men receiving honours for service in equine communities. Ads showed men in law, financial services, real estate, or with trucks. There were a few images that were notably different:

men at a healing centre, two toddlers with horses, and two family members with a woman adopting a horse.

Almost every grown man shown in the photographs in this catalogue was professionally involved with horses. The women's roles included competitive riding and a few pictures representing careers as veterinary assistants, coaches, and chiropractors, but most pictures of women with horses showed no hint of a horse career. And there were several images of women cuddling horses or kissing their noses.

Does this match your experience? Do you like to just *be* with a horse, even if you don't make money or gain status or accomplish some useful task such as pulling logs or rounding up cattle? If so, what is that relationship about (assuming Desmond Morris didn't have the whole picture)? Subjective feelings cannot be explained objectively, but in *The Tao of Equus*, Linda Kohanov tries to describe the experience of the woman-horse bond. She says it is as if they've resurrected a lost part of themselves while galloping down the trail, as if all the centuries that men went to war on well-trained steeds seem trivial compared to a single moment of understanding between a teenage girl and her first bay mare."

I often wonder if women in the modern Western world crave something of the horse's way of being. I recall working in an organization where executives sought out and valued my perspectives (though I'm not so sure about the middle managers). If you know the Myers-Briggs personality assessment tool often used in organizations, my preferences are "INTP." The details of those preferences aren't important for this story. What is important is that they are relatively uncommon in our society and very uncommon in the organization where I worked. So I concluded: "I think differently than most people here, and the executives find me helpful because I bring in new perspectives." That may have been true, but a few years later, when I worked with gender issues in education, I decided my value might simply have been as a woman who cared about things such as context and relationship, in a male organization where that was rare. Sadly, I remember feeling a bit disappointed about that!

In our careers, I have noticed that my colleagues and I were usually rewarded for being strategic, calculating (not necessarily in a bad way), logical, linear, sequential, and unemotional: traits typically valued by men. I recall watching a televised debrief of a national political debate in which an announcer postulated that our prime minister had won the debate (about very significant issues) because he didn't show any emotion. Intuition is rarely rewarded, unless it is backed by analysis. The ability to read body language isn't listed in many job descriptions. Observations about the present moment are distractions in the quest for a more profitable or effective future. But when we interact with horses, the experience is in the moment and very different. As Allan Hamilton puts it: "Horses seem to come along at the right time with the right things to teach us." Perhaps horses help us transition from the decades of coping with workplace cultures that are very different from the culture of horses.

In our family lives, women, at least in my generation, are famous for putting other people's needs and schedules ahead of our own. We almost forget how to live in the moment. I have heard many women say that when their husbands travel, it takes them a few days to really get in touch with what they want to do. Horses do little strategizing. They are masterful readers of the world around them and the moment is all-important. We humans often position ourselves as better than other animals because of our strategic and analytical skills. If horses were the ones to develop IQ tests, I think most humans would have severe intellectual disabilities.

I was grooming Bocina one day, and I was a bit tense and "in my head" rather than in my heart (as I often am). I remembered things I had read about being in tune with your horse. I stopped grooming her, stood by her head, and began to breathe very slowly and deeply. She turned towards me slightly and within a few seconds she was matching my breathing. These moments between us don't yet happen often, but I am so moved when they do. I hope they will become common.

Always keep in mind that relationships take time and effort to build. Don't feel frustrated at six months or a year or five years because you aren't quite "there" yet. In *Zen Mind, Zen Horse*, Allan Hamilton reminds us that, at the end of his life, Michelangelo stated: "I am dying just as I begin to learn the alphabet of my profession."

POINTS TO PONDER

▶ Understanding and relationship building take time, and there isn't a recipe book for success.

▶ Most people involved with horses are women, and they don't necessarily get involved with specific goals, such as a career or competition.

▶ We are only beginning to understand woman-horse relationships; they seem diverse and multi-layered. Women describe these relationships in many different ways, often using language that is more intuitive than scientific.

QUESTION TO CONSIDER

▶ How might you develop calmness and patience in working with your horse? What activities might help you do this? Grooming your horse? Sitting in their field without expectations?

"When I bestride him, I soar, I am a hawk.
He trots the air, the earth sings when he touches it."
WILLIAM SHAKESPEARE

9 | Learning to Speak Horse: The C Words

WHAT WILL BE the nature of the relationship you develop with your horse? There are many "flavours," especially in relation to leadership. What vehicles or languages will you choose to enhance communication between you and your horse? How do things like energy play into this learning?

There is a paradox here as we contemplate the meaning of "relationship" in ways that may not fit with our logical, linear, cerebral upbringings. I share some heady ideas, including chi, morphic resonance, and subtle body language, because you may find them fascinating threads that weave through your evolving relationship with your horse. At the same time, they can get your brain working in overdrive, which pulls you away from the emotional and somatic elements of relationship we are exploring. And you thought raising teenagers was complex!

This is a chapter for sipping. If the first part of the book was a bit like "how to change a tire." Learning to speak horse is more like "how to fit into a new culture." The content is complex, contextual, and maybe even controversial. *There is no recipe book; there are no generic right answers.* Many horse people will tell you that the search for answers constantly reveals interesting questions.

I draw on the thinking of many diverse people here because I believe their insights will be valuable for you at various times during this learning journey. Some of you will find the ideas here fascinating, some may find it less useful than the practical tips, and some may find it to be like a smorgasbord: you keep coming back for different servings of this buffet of ideas.

C Words and Leadership

As you build your relationship with your horse, you will find yourself thinking about control, compliance, communication, connection, care and compassion, cooperation, collaboration, and even chi. Of course, these are all related to the L word: leadership. These C words are vocabulary in the language of relationship building with your horse. The ones you choose to focus on will affect the principles behind how you interact with your horse and how the relationship evolves.

I work professionally with leadership development. "Leadership" is one of those words that we use as though we understand what others mean when they use it. In our Western culture, we often assume leader = person = adult = male = man with a job title that tells you he must be a leader (president, CEO, director).

You have undoubtedly heard that a horse—as a prey animal—needs a strong leader in order to thrive. The "prey animal" part of this is key. Most people in this twenty-first-century culture have more experience with dogs than horses. Like humans, dogs are predators. When they face a potential threat, dogs and humans have fight-or-flight options, as well as abilities to work with strategies and tactics. When threatened, a horse only wants to flee. If your horse is confident in you as a leader, she can relax and not worry so much about survival or about all the responsibilities associated with protecting the herd. But what does that really mean?

If we apply the boss-equals-leader model of leadership, we could assume leadership is based on *communication*, *control*, and *compliance*. You decide what needs to be done, you tell your horse what to do, you firmly insist on certain responses—and your horse complies. It is clear that you are the boss. Your horse trusts you to be the boss and does exactly what you say. He respects your personal space. He backs up when you ask. He lifts each hoof in turn to be cleaned. However, if you have had a career outside the home, you know that compliant employees aren't great employees. If their workday ends at 4:30, they are out the door at 4:31. If they are expected to do good work, they do not strive for excellence. If they have to make decisions without your direction, they may struggle.

So do we want control and compliance with our horses? To a degree we do. And perhaps that is precisely what some people want. But for the rest of us, how do we determine whether our horses are simply complying in a joyless and unimaginative kind of way? Other than saying that observation and intuition are involved, I do not yet have answers and I struggle with this.

Alexandra Hamilton, my farrier, is an experienced horse-woman and I hope to develop half her sensitivity over time.

One of her horses is a massive 17.3-hand solid black Olden-burg mare named Tarot. I haven't seen their relationship first-hand but have heard about it from several angles. A friend described seeing them on the Trans Canada Trail: Alex who is a solid, strikingly beautiful woman with long black hair was cantering bareback with a halter on this huge black horse. My friend isn't easily impressed, but she was clearly moved by the image. As a younger horse, Tarot had done a lot of showing and travelling, but Alex said it was just too much for her.

Tarot needed to be in a safe, stable place where her feelings mattered. Alex realized that Tarot hated the ring, but together they discovered her passion for the trails. Tarot was brave and strong and energetic, and as Alex put it, "the ground we covered and the times she saved my butt!!"

I contacted Alex about details of this story and got an interesting update. Tarot is a "roarer," a term used to describe horses with breathing problems, especially when exercising. An inhalation sounds like a harsh roar. Alex knew it was time for either retirement or surgery, and she felt she owed Tarot the latter. So they went ahead with the surgery and rehab, and now Tarot is as fit as ever. However, when Alex goes out in the field with the intention of riding, Tarot chooses to step back and mind the fort while Alex takes another horse out. She is sweeter than ever, but doesn't want to go out. Alex has let Tarot decide what much of their relationship looks like, a brilliant example of shared leadership. It hasn't always been smooth sailing: "I love her to bits, though we clash and have personalities oh so similar that catch me quite often reflecting back to myself," says Alex. Looking ahead, Alex thinks Tarot will want to ride again, but if that day doesn't come, she says, "I can still smile about the wings she gave me."

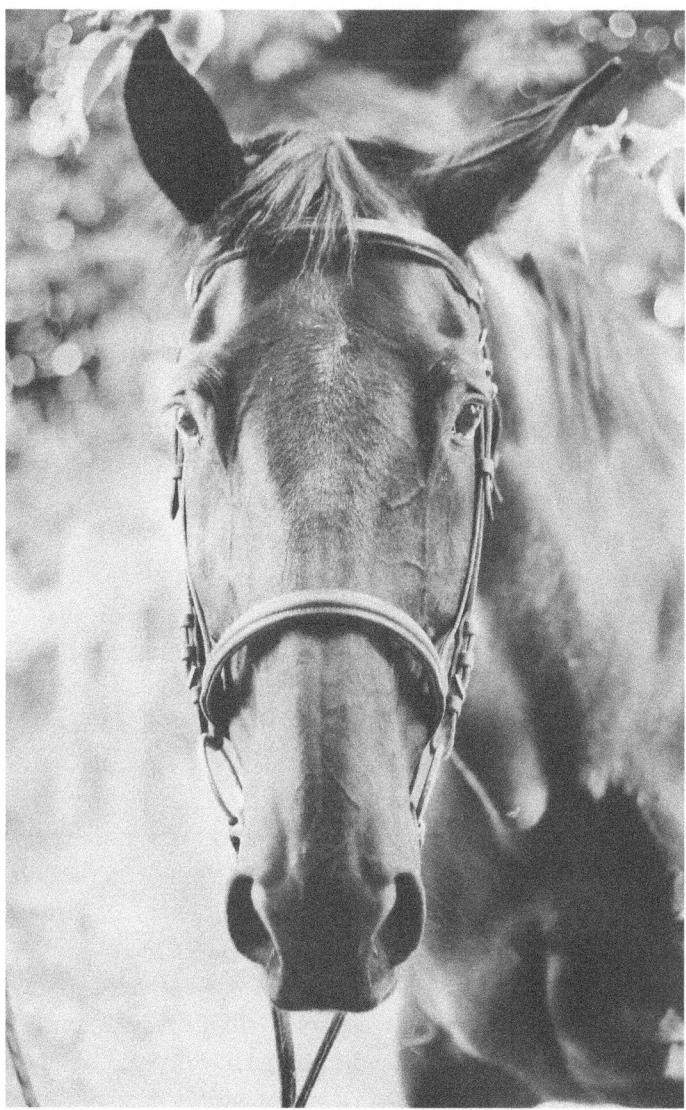

ABOVE *Tarot has had ups and downs in her life. On this day, her worries were palpable.* Photo: AMANDA EDWARDS PHOTOGRAPHY

When Alex said that, I pictured them as a single being, a sort of Pegasus. Perhaps that is the feeling my friend had when she first saw them on the trail. I often think about and aspire to this sort of horse-human hybrid being. And then I learned more through feminist scholar Donna Haraway's work, in which she cites Jean-Claude Barry, who studied unintentional movements by skilled riders: "Muscles fire and contract in both horse and human at precisely the same time." In other words, the two are supremely tuned to each other; it is no longer clear where the signals start or end. Alex shared something about her ever-evolving relationship with Tarot that we could all take to heart: "I feel blessed I am able to consider the mental well being of the animals in my family." Such is the nature of relationship building.

Looking back at people and organizations, there are many types of leadership theories that have nothing to do with command and control. Their names are descriptive: "distributed," "shared," "relational," and "complex." These theories all get away from the charismatic and heroic leader who sees the future and directs the way. In my work with organizations, I usually find these theories more helpful and more attractive than command-and-control models.

As one example, I researched a successful community of scientists and first responders who had come together voluntarily from several organizations. There was a coordinator of sorts, but he said he definitely wasn't the leader. He described how everyone in the group was a leader and how impressed he was by their leadership. In his regular job as a senior manager, he really had to keep tabs on people and be sure work was being done. However, with the community group, he said that when it was quiet, he knew good things were happening. Everyone else in the group spoke about him as a leader they really respected. When I asked them about what he did to gain their respect, most of them mentioned his understanding of the field and his ability to connect people who didn't know each other at just the right time. He put a lot of effort into *context* and *connections*, and he made a space in which people could feel respected. He wanted them to learn, grow, and thrive in a healthy, unconstrained way.

As another example, I spent time with an American police department where they had developed an unusual leadership model. Police departments are known for a command-and-control culture, and police chiefs have moved up through that system. In this Oklahoma town, all the important policy decisions had been delegated to a diverse group of sworn and civilian members from all levels of the department. People *loved* working there. They designed innovative programs for the public. One time the chief of police was in town and the fire chief came up to him and said, "I love that new program for seniors you've put together." "Oh, which one is that?" Chief Wuestewald asked. "Oh, the one where your guys and my guys go into the homes and check smoke alarms and security, etc. The seniors love it. It is working so well, and I am sure we have prevented some fires." What the police chief didn't reveal was that he was totally unaware of that program at the time; the climate that grew out of shared leadership naturally evolved into people taking initiative. The model was strongly *collaborative*.

But are collaborative models appropriate for work with a prey species? Perhaps a story from near my home will help turn our thinking on its side. Was the work of setting up innovative programs for seniors that much different—in spirit—from the behaviour of Irish, my friend Maggie's Rocky Mountain Horse? Maggie, her friend Kelly, and their horses were hanging out in a field enjoying themselves, when Irish left Maggie's side and walked away. Maggie was a bit disappointed until she looked over to see Irish by a wooden platform the horses were sometimes asked to step onto. There was Irish with his front feet on the platform, looking very pleased with himself and delighted that Maggie had discovered him there. Yes, his reward from her pocket was less sophisticated than great public feedback to the police department, but Irish had taken unexpected initiative, or dare we say *leadership*? Was he training his human?

In her book *Dressage with Mind, Body, and Soul*, Linda Tellington-Jones suggests you want your horse to act like "an intelligent, independent being who is capable of taking care of you in certain situations, not just vice versa." In the documentary *Sur la Voie du Cheval*, Mark Rashid speaks about horses in the wild:

> The boss in the herd can be referred to as the Alpha Horse. And a lot of people refer to that as the one we want to emulate. If you've ever spent any time around any large herds of horses it's real easy to find the alpha horse—the boss horse. Because they are generally off by themselves, because the other horses just don't want to be around them. So for me, I don't know why we want to emulate that behaviour in relation to training and working with horses.

Mark goes on to describe how there is also a leader, separate from the boss. This is usually an older mare who is trusted and knowledgeable. I find it interesting how these human terms—"boss" and "leader"—are applied to the herd. In our workplaces, we have all met bosses who clawed their way to the top, and their paycheques are bigger than their circles of workplace friends. And we have all met leaders who can be anywhere in an organization and you would never quickly spot them from the outside.

Horseman Mark Bolender believes collaborative models are essential for safe, effective work with horses. He may not have studied leadership theory, but he describes his philosophy in a leadership frame: "Good horsemanship is not about domination but leadership, and having the horse volunteer for a partnership with the handler." This echoes ideas from shared and distributed leadership, and perhaps even from complex leadership, where leadership can *emerge* from the space in between.

Feminist scholar Donna Haraway goes further when she criticizes perceptions of cross-species relationships in dog agility work. In *Where Species Meet*, Haraway states that the term "handler" implies that "human agility partners imagine they have their controlling hands on the helm of nature." While we're on this topic of language, I increasingly wrestle with the term horse "owner." There are things I like about it. If I ever mistreated my mare and the SPCA came to get her, I think it should be absolutely clear that I am the one responsible for her care and the one who should be punished for the mistreatment. But other things about the term bother me. Gayle Ecker, the director of Equine Guelph, told me, "I own my tractor, but that doesn't mean I take care of it." She prefers the term "caretaker" to "owner." "Steward" is another term that is more balanced than "owner." Given that our society considers non-human animals inferior, it isn't surprising that we have to hunt for a word that conveys elements of partnership, parenting, care, and leadership between humans and other animals.

Mark Bolender is skilled in several disciplines and special-izes in mountain trail, extreme trail, and competitive trail pur-suits. In his clinics, riders and handlers are given instructions with a focus on helping the horses become calm, confident, and skilled as they encounter new types of obstacles. Once in a clinic I saw him holding the rope of a participant's horse. The horse had a front hoof on a wooden bridge and his back hooves on the arena footing. This was progress. Mark spoke to the audience for a long time, appearing to ignore the horse, who stood essentially motionless. Mark realized audience members were probably puzzled by the lack of aids and he said: "I like to have them learn from their own decisions." This does not sound like *communication, control* and *compliance*; it is more like *collaboration*. Of course, clinicians like Mark "speak horse" so fluently that they have become unconsciously com-petent. We can learn as much from watching them over time as we do from hearing their human language words.

Enhanced Communication

Communication between you and your horse can be enhanced (or diminished) through riding. Dressage and rein-ing are two disciplines requiring superb communication between horse and rider. There are several videos and good information about both on the web. There is even a video showing both disciplines demonstrated together. Because I ride English, and because dressage is more common than reining, I will only speak to dressage.

Dressage sometimes gets a bad rap. Most dressage you would stumble upon on television is at an international competition level in which the skills are extreme. At these high levels, the moves may not seem useful (and perhaps boring to those who do not ride, though some people are intrigued by the way the elite horses "dance"). I have heard

TV announcers joke about watching dressage being like "watching paint dry." But if you are new to dressage and carefully observe a Grand Prix performance, you will see incredibly subtle communication. A good dressage rider's hands are almost motionless. If you "speak horse" well, you will notice the communication is very much two-way. Dressage (which simply means "training" in French) can be a language through which you learn to speak across the species barrier.

If you are reading this book you probably have no international competition goals. Why would you consider dressage (or reining in the Western world), if your passions lie in trail riding, driving, or just hanging out with your horse? Because cross-training with dressage has many benefits. Equine Canada describes the purpose of dressage as "designed to improve a horse's balance, suppleness and flexibility, as well as improve the communication between horse and rider." The United States Equestrian Federation states dressage is for "the harmonious development of the physique and ability of a horse." Dressage expert and author Jane Savoie explains how dressage has many purposes, including the extension of your horse's functional years, provision of "physiotherapy" for a variety of horse body issues, athletic conditioning of the horse, helping a shy horse gain confidence, provision of a medium where learning can be wonderful for both of you, and enhancement of the *communication* and *cooperation* between horse and rider. Jane Savoie emphasizes kindness as an underlying principle of dressage training, as well as two more C words: *clarity* and *consistency*. When I rode a bit as a teen, I didn't understand any of this. And I have spoken to many women who were casual Western riders, and this idea of taking your horse to the gym was foreign to them, too. The skills are not ones horses develop on their own, out in the pasture.

The first summer I had my mare, I rode over to watch a local fun event (because I mistakenly thought I wasn't yet good enough to participate). The women were in my age range, though they had more experience with horses than I did. There were ten games with points attached to each. In one, Kerry—an experienced Western rider—bent over to pick up a flag. Her horse, Shilo, bolted. Kerry got him under control quickly and reassured him. A few months later, Deborah Fox—a superb dressage coach—started to come to our island on Sundays. When she first saw Shilo walk around the ring, she said: "With this horse, it's all about balance; if we don't get him balanced, there will be problems." I couldn't see the balance issues but remembered the flag incident. As Kerry and Shilo started dressage training, I could clearly see changes. Within a few months, Shilo looked years younger. And both Kerry and Shilo loved the communication and growth. "He gets it," Kerry said of the dressage work. "It's like taking your horse to the gym." After several months of consistent work in the dressage ring and on the lunge line, the coach suggested Kerry register Shilo in a legitimate show with a high-level judge. Kerry and Shilo took the top ribbons in their category.

I had an interesting experience in a recent dressage lesson. Deborah, who normally gives specific directions to improve technique, suggested I was thinking too much. She was right (although I have not yet figured out how to consistently ride properly using more intuition and less linear thinking). At one point, she said something like "just touch with your outside leg and visualize the curve." It worked beautifully. This got me thinking about ideas Linda Tellington-Jones has shared about a new foundation for dressage training. She tells a story from the last clinic taught by dressage Olympian Reiner Klimke before he passed away. Participants had to enter the arena on the proper path at a trot, with a loose rein. Most of the talented riders found this very difficult, and some found it impossible. The horses were used to a lot of detailed guidance. This was one instance that got Linda thinking about what is missing in dressage training. She uses colour metaphors as a way to develop a more solid, balanced foundation for the steps of dressage training. I offer this simply as an example of how the things you encounter may at first seem strange, foreign, or uncomfortable, but that discomfort may be a good indicator that this new learning might be especially powerful. Consider the Chinese proverb: "Be not afraid of growing slowly. Be afraid only of standing still."

I quickly learned that my traditional education (simply from living in this culture as well as formal education) did not prepare me well for communication with a horse. I needed to look to other fields and other cultures. Allan Hamilton—renowned horse trainer and Harvard-educated brain surgeon—was the first person I encountered who made an explicit connection between chi and work with horses. Like most North Americans, I have a superficial understanding of chi from martial arts documentaries, some tai chi classes, and conversations about Chinese medicine. I am not qualified to sum up its essence. It might be translated as "life force," or "energy flow." We seem to think of energy very differently in the Western and Eastern worlds. The chi, or qi, concept goes beyond the boundaries of a body or a lifetime. Chi is tied to intention: a familiar concept for horsewomen. Hamilton describes an experiment to demonstrate chi. He suggests you sit in a pasture with horses for some time, and then walk towards the grazing group, directing your energy towards a specific horse you plan to halter. Typically, the horse you have chosen will react while the others seem oblivious.

There are varied ways of understanding such communication with horses, which may be interrelated, different interpretations of the same phenomenon, or separate phenomena. In addition to chi, one is morphic resonance and another is extreme sensitivity to body language.

Rupert Sheldrake developed the idea of morphic resonance. I first saw Sheldrake on a twelve-part PBS special many years ago. I was fascinated by his research and equally fascinated by the way that other experts on the program seemed almost angry about his research. Sheldrake has impressive academic credentials: he was a Fellow of Clare College, Cambridge, where he was director of studies in biochemistry and cell biology. However, conclusions from some of his research were far enough outside the accepted tenets of Western science that he was pushed (or pulled) into more independent studies. He often works with people and their pets, because costs are low and the animals are treated more kindly than are lab animals. His experiments are fun and simple, and pet owners can take part with little or no cost.

Central to much of Sheldrake's work is the idea that *the mind is larger than the brain,* so the mind can therefore influence things at a distance. There is no evidence the brain and mind are the same size and shape, yet most of us embraced this assumption, perhaps based on an elementary school teacher's description of a textbook graphic. If our minds are much larger than we are, it makes sense that creatures close to us for whatever reason—you and your horse, for example—might meaningfully connect in the physical space between you, whether that be a few feet or many miles. Hamilton's experiment with haltering a horse might also be explained using different terms. For example, your mind extends out to the horse in question, and as a sensitive prey species, the horse has the experience of being stared at. I have seen Sheldrake present research in a time-coded, split-screen video format where a pet owner is in one location and the pet in the other. The scientific evidence clearly shows communication between owner and pet as a research assistant takes the owner home in a taxi while the dog increasingly anticipates her arrival. Sheldrake's website is also full of in-depth resources for the intellectually curious. It lists his books, including his very accessible volume: *Dogs That Know When Their Owners Are Coming Home.*

Body language is also a huge part of equine-human communication. Tellington-Jones writes about one tiny element of this body language: nibbles and biting. She says,

> when your horse tries to bite, nip, lip, pinch or even nibble on you, he is giving you an important piece of communication. When simply "lipping" or licking you, I believe he is transmitting friendliness and a desire for attention; if you are a horse with four feet on the ground, what do you have? Your mouth! Then there are the playful nips, such as when foals think they can treat you like another horse: they haven't yet learned the distinction between foals and people.
>
> A horse who snaps at the air is trying to tell you that he is nervous about the way he is groomed or the girth is tightened, or his back is sore, or he is exceedingly sensitive and can't take what you are doing. His whispers have failed and the biting is the "shout."

You may have heard about the famous German horse of the early 1900s who appeared to have extraordinary abilities. Clever Hans—as he came to be known—would answer quite complicated questions by tapping his hoof. Clever Hans and his owner, Wilhelm von Osten, attracted such attention

that there were scientific studies conducted to better understand just what was going on. If his handler did not know
the answers, the horse would not reliably provide correct
answers. Clever Hans also "lost his abilities" when he could
not see the person asking the questions. People *unconsciously*
cued him (this was considered to be a "peculiarly interesting feature of the case") about when to stop tapping his hoof.
In her book *Smart Horse*, Jennifer MacLeay states that the
unconscious raising of the handler's eyebrows was the trigger of acceptance or recognition that signalled Clever Hans
to stop tapping. Others have suggested a lifting of the head,
flaring of nostrils, or change in stance would trigger the horse
in similar ways. Regardless, the story of Clever Hans illustrates how horses can read the subtlest of cues.

There is no point trying to disguise an emotion around
your horse. Sometimes if I can't shake a negative emotion,
I talk to my horse about it. I know she doesn't understand
the words, but it helps me to be in the moment and aware of
what is going on with my energy. She really pays attention
when we have these "conversations."

These ideas of subtle cues through mind, body language,
and energy relate strongly to *communication* and *connection*. If
these ideas intrigue you, I suggest you read Allan Hamilton's
book *Zen Mind, Zen Horse: The Science and Spirituality of Working
with Horses* as a starting point. It complements other good
horse books by digging deeply into what we have become as
humans, what horses have become, and the little-understood
territory in the middle. The practical tips in it are steeped in
context. Perhaps you are a cook who constantly creates reci-
pes because you understand different ingredients and how
they interact? Perhaps your neighbour cannot make pancakes without a mix? Her pancakes might taste fine, but she

has constraints that you have overcome. I think it is the same with horsemanship. Some people probably handle horses in a pancake-mix kind of way: 1) Hold the outside rein firmly; 2) Add some right leg; 3) Vibrate the left rein, and there you have it. Period. They might not want to think about brain science, predator-prey relations, ritual, or chi. If you like to dig deep, if you are drawn to questions like "why" and "what if" as much as "how," Hamilton's book is one you are apt to browse for years.

Finally, it's important to emphasize that horses have very good senses, including smell, hearing, and sight. I often wonder if horses, as prey animals, react to vegetarian humans differently than meat-eating ones. Horses have large eyes and excellent vision in almost all directions and even in dim light. They can see colour, though not with the detail of the human eye. Your horse recognizes your voice and your face, even if you have been away for some time. NBC news reported research by ethologist Carol Sankey and her colleagues about how horses in France remembered a female trainer and her instructions after a separation of up to eight months. In another study, Sherril Stone, a researcher from Oklahoma State University, used photographs to explore whether horses recognized individual people even in two-dimensional images and found that they do. Some ideas for the application of her findings are to "introduce" human clients to therapy horses before they meet by showing pictures to the horses (and perhaps clients) or to put a picture of yourself where your horse can see it in your absence.

Find a Translator

There are cross-cultural communication specialists all over the world, helping people to understand and work with each

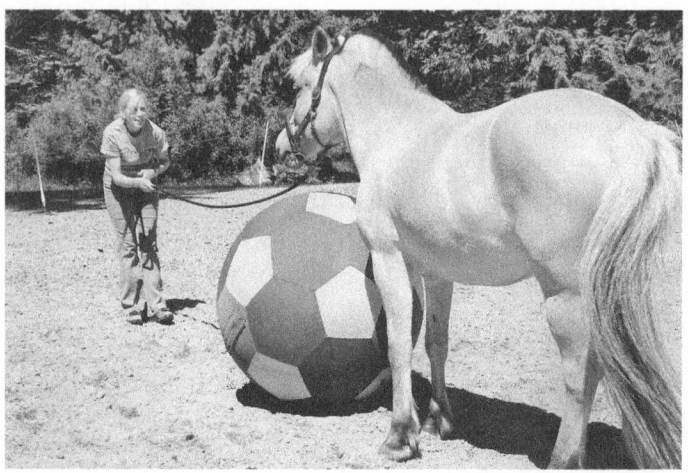

ABOVE *Kelly Bilquist tries to convince Bocina that a hoof ball can be great fun.* Photo: ALICE MACGILLIVRAY

other across national, religious, ethnic, and cultural boundaries. Yet we are all human beings. It should be relatively simple. But getting humans and horses to understand each other is more like getting wolves and sheep to understand each other. We can learn a lot by bringing somewhat bilingual translators into our lives.

When our relationship was very new, I took Bocina to a friend's property. Kelly's property is fun; riders often have problems getting past it, as the horses associate it with good experiences. Kelly had arranged a course on equine massage and there were about six horses of as many breeds there, with people trying out their new skills. Bocina likes the geldings who live on that property and, though behaving well, was being a bit of a flirt. Then another woman walked over leading a retired Fjord gelding. I instantly thought of those Japanese music videos where a young man and woman run across soft-focus pastel fields in slow motion. The world disappeared around the two Fjords as they met each other and sniffed each other's faces. I don't recall Kelly's exact commentary, but it went something like this:

Kelly: Now they're going to squeal.

(Alice thinks: Squeal? What's a squeal? I thought they liked each other, why would they squeal? Yikes—that's a squeal? So glad I knew it was coming; would have scared the heck out of me.)

Kelly: Oh, they're going to do the neck wrap! Awwww.

(Alice thinks: What's a neck wrap? Oh—that's a neck wrap. That's cute—they've buried their noses in each other's necks, and look at those deep breaths. Wow. How did she know that was coming?)

This commentary went on with Kelly anticipating the language and my being able to study it as it unfolded. You can't have enough ways of learning when you want to speak horse.

Consider keeping a journal. If you have ever learned a second or third language, you know the learning sneaks up on you. There are awkward periods, plateaux, and breakthroughs. Sometimes you feel like a beginner, and the next thing you know, you have a dream in the new language. If you journal about the learning—perhaps with sketches of horse body language—you will have documented milestones to celebrate.

POINTS TO PONDER

▸ The intelligence of horses is different from human intelligence.

▸ There are many ways to think about leadership; they aren't all about leaders as bosses. If you work with leadership in human systems, see what you can learn from your horse that might be transferable.

▶ Listen to opinions and advice, but don't expect to find a recipe book for leading or communicating with your horse.

▶ Think about what you want in your human-horse relationship and how important it is for you to move beyond compliance.

▶ Find ways of helping your horse learn from his own decisions.

▶ Consider dressage as a way of building communication between you and your horse.

▶ Be willing to set aside your knowledge of communication as a rational act. Be open to practising work with chi and other concepts that may be new to you.

▶ Horses are master readers of body language; don't try to fool them.

▶ Spend time with people such as good coaches who speak horse fluently and learn from them.

▶ Consider keeping a journal to record how your ability to speak horse evolves over time.

QUESTION TO CONSIDER

▶ Which C words appeal most to you? How might emphasis on those ideas influence your relationship with your horse?

10 | Learning to Speak Equestrian

DURING MY FIRST two years of horse owner-
ship, I often expressed frustration about how horse gear sup-
pliers assume customers speak fluent equestrian. A vendor's
website section about horse "clothing" might list turnout
blankets, rain sheets, stable blankets, quarter sheets, open
front sheets, exercise rugs, blanket liners, and other products
with no descriptions of purpose. A section about horse boots
might include bell boots, specialty boots, open-front boots,
simple boots, and ankle boots. You could tell that "shipping boots" were presumably for shipping, but "bell boots"
wouldn't be for bells. So, I started a glossary to include in
this book. Days later, a new catalogue from a major company
arrived in my mailbox, with contextual text for each product *category*. In the hope that this is a trend, I set the glossary
aside. But product category descriptions may not help you
much with decisions such as "What should my horse wear

while being trailered to my property?" or "Should I buy polo wraps as part of the standard kit for my horse?"

Of course, equestrian-speak goes well beyond tack. How does a pasture compare with a paddock? What is free lease? Self-board? Having your horse light versus soft? What does "grain" mean? (I thought I knew.) What are good bloodlines and breeding for a particular horse? You overhear someone ask "Is that driving dressage, pleasure driving, or CDE?" (Thankfully, you don't have to answer). And what do you do when you're trying out your first horse and her owner asks you to do a half-halt?

Some of the ways to cope with the flood of equestrian terminology are to:

1. Realize it comes with the territory; don't be intimidated, and see it as an opportunity to learn.
2. Concentrate on high priorities, such as safety for you and the horse and optimal nutrition.
3. Ask lots of conversation-generating questions, such as:
   a. What do you mean by that?
   b. Why is that important?
   c. Someone else suggested... Could you say more?
   d. Do you have a picture or could you show me?
   e. Why do you prefer that?
   f. What sorts of risks are there?
   g. Where could I learn more?
4. Realize there are many specialized sources of expertise. For example, if your horse is being shipped over a long distance, a good horse-hauling company will know more about what she should wear than a tack shop would. A veterinary college will know more about the latest deworming research than your favourite salesperson at the feed store.

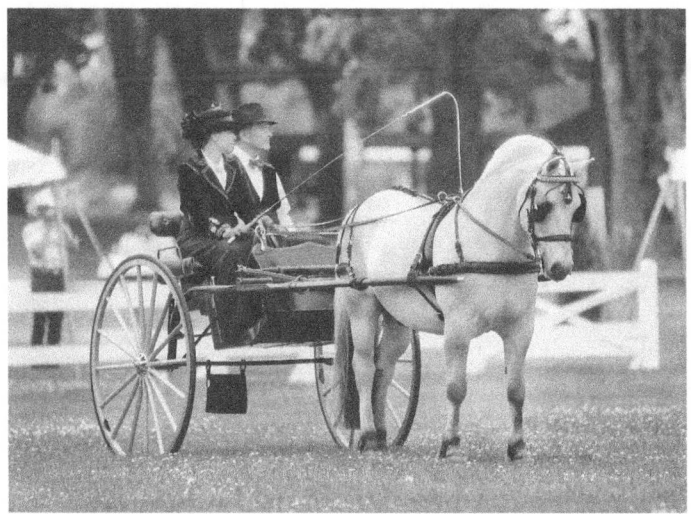

ABOVE *Peggy and her dad driving Prisco in the Father's Day Class. Partici-pating in this pleasure driving class was a highlight for Peggy's father.* Photo: JOEL PEREGRINE

5. Read and listen. If you have good Internet access, there are many superb resources. As I write this, a Google search of "What are side reins?" retrieves a massive number of links, including definitions, how-to videos, and warnings about their use. Pick up catalogues in tack shops. Subscribe to magazines you find valuable. Borrow books from the library and buy the ones you find most helpful. Go to clinics and trade shows. Listen to experienced people and ask open-ended questions.

6. Be patient and humble. Taking a weekend course on hoof trimming does not make you a farrier. Reading everything you can find about how to fit a saddle does not make you a saddle fitter. Claim expertise too soon, and you may provide your neighbours with some good chuckles.

Your Coach as a Translator

I cannot say enough about how important and wonderful it is to have a good coach. If, for whatever reason, you would not be able to have a good coach at least for your first few years of horse ownership, I would recommend you not get a horse.

There are certification programs for coaches, and the certifications have both disciplines and levels. If a coach is certified, you are presumably assured that they are competent, professional, and have demonstrated knowledge of such things as riding, ethics, coaching theory, and first aid. Coaches specialize to varying degrees. Some may work only with riders who don't want to compete or only with those who are competitive. Some may only coach Western. Some may offer a range of options, such as hunter/jumper and eventing, or English and dressage. In most cases, coaches help you to ride, but you will find some who focus on things such as driving, groundwork, or natural horsemanship. If they are associated with a facility, the facility website probably lists the specializations and levels of their coaches. If you're a beginner, I recommend you start with a certified coach, because you probably don't yet have the skills to judge coaching quality for you and your horse. However, there are also some great uncertified coaches out there, and you may find yourself working with some as you learn more.

Coaches coach you. They don't take your horse away and teach your horse to do things (unless you hire them as trainers). A really good coach has a lot of experience with horses and a great eye for quickly seeing the person/horse dynamic. They work from a vast base of tacit knowledge and know that every day and every lesson can be somewhat different for you and your horse. Your coach may occasionally hop on your horse, especially when you begin to work together. The coach then learns how much your horse knows (and doesn't know) and how well he responds to aids. Your horse may be a bit stiff in some part of his body. He may be nervous about the crows in the bushes or because he is picking up on your anxiety. As you ride, small body movements can make a huge difference. A good coach will notice that your outside shoulder isn't quite as far back as it was on the last corner or that you brought your inside rein back a bit as you started the circle. You get instant feedback on things you might not notice yourself, so you can see how good technique changes results.

A coach helps you to learn to speak equestrian in many ways. They will naturally use a lot of terminology. When they use terms you don't know (or that you only know in a superficial way from reading), they provide great opportunities for learning. You aren't just learning the terms. For example, if they ask you to use your "diagonal aids" of inside leg and outside rein, even if you know which leg is inside the which rein is outside, it takes a while to get the feel of how to do this and how to get your horse comfortable and understanding what you are "saying" to him. When you get it, you not only know the terms. You know the feel in your body and the feel of when everything is working well in your horse's body. When you accidentally steer a bit with the inside rein and you hear that your horse is losing balance, you absorb what that feels like, reestablish the feel of the firm outside rein, and rediscover the feel of your balanced horse. A good coach will be patient with you. Don't confuse assertive, repeated direction with impatience. If a coach needs to tell you something fifteen times in a lesson in a loud enough voice so that you can hear, she is probably also extremely supportive and patient. It takes a while to process the many things you need to think about as you are learning to ride well.

I want to briefly talk about the difference between a horse in a pasture and a horse with a rider. There are many good books that describe this in more detail. But understanding the basics is an important part of understanding why I think coaches are so important. Horses are designed to walk around and eat grass. Their bodies do this magnificently. They do whatever they need to do to maintain this ability. You might see them stretch occasionally, for example. Horses are not designed to walk around with one hundred (or two hundred) pounds on their backs. We came up with that idea and somehow talked them into it. They are remarkably cooperative about this. We can put on packs, saddles, riders, or saddlebags and they will head out onto the trail or wherever we ask them to go. They will walk around, just like they do in the field, but with all this extra weight.

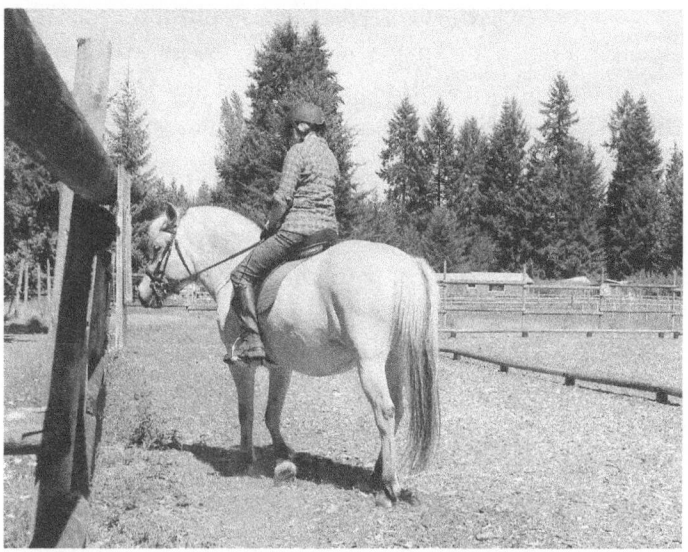

ABOVE Bonnie practises head-to-rail in a ring, keeping Bocina at a 30-degree angle to the fence. This sharpens the responsiveness of your horse so you can steer them quickly with leg aids as needed. Photo: ALICE MACGILLIVRAY

Have you ever gone on a backpacking trip without any preparation? You strap on the fifty-pound pack and it feels okay at first, but then you find yourself trying to shift the weight or use different muscles and you end up with back spasms. If you've had this experience, you've probably learned to get a really good-fitting pack and how to use core muscles and which machines at the gym help you to build those muscles. And you've probably gradually built up the strength so that you are comfortable and confident carrying the fifty-pound pack. An expert coach can look at a horse and see whether the owner just "throws on the pack" or whether the horse has been ridden to gradually build up the muscles and posture needed to carry a load comfortably and safely without compromising his body. When they build these muscles, carry their backs high, with their necks rounded, and they connect well with the bit, it is called longitudinal suppleness. Based on my experience, even if your horse knows how to do this, you need to learn as well. A coach becomes a sort of personal trainer for you and your horse, helping you to understand the terms and techniques that will help keep you both strong and healthy.

If you are lucky enough to have a choice of several good coaches, try them out. Give each one a chance. If you are concerned about something, talk with the coach to explore the problem. Perhaps you feel that you can't do anything right, but the coach tells you that you are doing amazingly well and they are providing specific feedback so that you can continue to improve. If the relationship with you, your horse, and your coach just isn't working after serious effort on your part, find another coach. In a pinch, you can learn from videos and the odd trip to a clinic. But keep learning. This is one of the great joys of becoming a horse owner.

Risks of Not Knowing

Perhaps the biggest thing to realize is how much you don't know. With me, it was often the basics. For example, when I saw a property listed with a riding ring my typical reaction was "Sounds like work, and rings would be for *competitive* riders." Now I would love to have quick access to a good ring. A ring is a great place for relatively safe, structured practice. I see women who have worked and learned with horses all their lives who are constantly moving into some new area of learning where they realize how little they know.

The diagram showing relationships between knowledge (what you know) and your perceptions of knowledge (what you realize you know) can be helpful for assessing risks. Here is how the categories, adapted from the Johari window, work:

1. I know how to have my horse leg-yield in a trot: I *know that I know* how to do a leg-yield.
2. We do not know how to do a half-pass; I *know that I don't know* how to do a half-pass.

   Sometimes the relationships between knowing and perceptions of knowing are more subtle and mysterious.
3. I might get a compliment about how I do something well, and I hadn't even realized I had that expertise: I *didn't know what I knew.*

   The risk increases with the final quadrant, where:
4. *You don't know that you don't know.* Sometimes the risk is low. I was helping a woman shop for a Fjord horse recently. I sent several website and video links and some breed facts. One message I sent said something like "I think this one is a steal." The horse was being sold because of owner health reasons. The sire and dam were among the most famous of all time in the country; the horse had considerable training from skilled

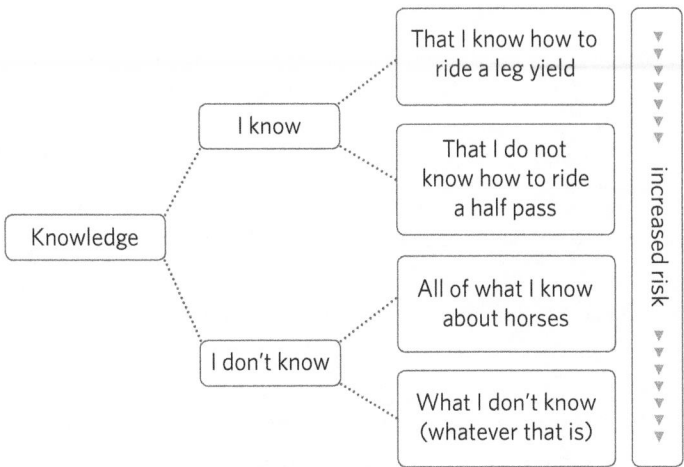

Figure 1: *A way of assessing your evolving knowledge*

trainers in more than one discipline, had shown successfully, and was healthy. The person wrote back: "Too old." The horse was fourteen. This might or might not have been the best horse for her, but she had drawn a mental line in the sand, probably based on longevity of other breeds.

Sometimes the risk is moderately higher. A friend horse-proofed her property over several years and then brought her first Fjord horses home. Here is part of her story:

> Fjords are way more industrious (and I dare I say intel-ligent) than other breeds. We had other horses here for 3 years before we got our first two Fjords, and within a day or two of arriving, the Fjords found all the "holes" in our facilities that were new and purpose-built and had worked just fine for our other horses.
>
> Door latches that had been just fine for three years, they opened and let themselves into the barn. Once

inside they took all of our stuff off the walls, threw it on the floor, and then walked on, chewed on, pooped on, and just generally vandalized everything! A rubber container with fence battery in it we used to have in the pasture and the horses just left it alone, well the Fjords opened it up, disconnected the battery and proceeded to carry it around by the strap on top (50 lb lead acid battery!).

Claudia, another Fjord owner, shared this memorable experience:

We have a long barn with a ground-level hay mow at one end, separated from the stall area by a Dutch door. We had just put in a second load of new hay, stacked quite high, but didn't have a gate to keep the horses out of it, so I had my car parked across the access to it, and of course the Dutch door was closed.

Inventive Vergel figured out how to open the Dutch door and jumped over the hood of my car. When I found him, he was about ten bales up on top of the pile, sorting around for the best hay. I yelled at him to get down. He looked at me with disgust at my spoiling his fun, but he obediently turned around, sat down on his fat rump and slid down to the ground, like a kid sliding down the stairs. I wouldn't have believed it if I hadn't found little Fjord hairs on my hood, traces of blue paint on Vergel's belly, and two neat dents in one fender... coincidentally the same distance apart as Vergel's feet.

Claudia used to have a big clever Morgan gelding named Spring. Early one year, Spring stayed at a boarding stable in Wisconsin for three weeks of extra riding and training. The only place left to keep him was called the "triangle," situated in the middle of several paddocks. Claudia explained:

> Each time I went to ride, he got hotter and harder to handle, and it got to the point where I approached the barn manager and asked how much they were feeding him. He said they were only feeding the small amount I had told them, and were as puzzled as I was about his wild behavior.
>
> Then one day I went there and the manager called me into the office, laughing, and said, "I figured out why your horse is so hot." The horses in the paddocks surrounding "the triangle" were fed in black rubber feed pans on the ground, as was Spring. The feeder would put the grain in their pans. All the black pans were tied to the fence posts with twine so the horses couldn't pick them up and toss them over the fences, etc. The barn manager said he watched while the feeder filled all the pans, including Spring's. Then Spring went around the perimeter of the triangle and pulled every feed pan into his own pen. There were six that he could reach in addition to his own. Apparently the horses whose grain he stole were not smart enough to pull the tubs back into their own enclosures, so they watched in frustration as Spring went from one tub to the next, consuming seven tubs of grain at each feeding. No one saw Spring steal the pans until Bill decided to watch carefully that day. After that, he watched two more times, to make sure it wasn't a fluke. It wasn't. Spring had it carefully figured out, and just *loved* feeding time, when he got to eat seven helpings! The funniest thing is that he didn't eat one, then go to the next; he pulled all of them into his triangle first, then ate.

As amusing as these stories are, these situations could have caused injury or illness for the horses or more serious property damage for the people.

Then there are the *really* close calls. Mae Mays got her first horse—a young, energetic mare named Star—when she was fifty-five. She bravely tackled horse trailering for the first time and managed to stay on Star when she kicked up her heels during their early rides. A woman suggested she lunge Star before riding but did not mention the importance of pacing and changes in direction. So after many circles in one direction, Star exploded. "She came at me with her mouth open and her teeth bared," Mae recalled. "I had a lunge whip and stood my ground, but she ripped the line out of my hand." Mae realized there was a serious problem and got good professional help without being injured.

I met another woman who had attended a four-day clinic with her horse. The clinician pulled her aside, explained she could no longer participate, and said her horse should be put down because he was dangerous: he had no respect for people on the ground. The woman was devastated and eventually found Sandy McMahon, a wonderful uncertified coach who helped them work through the respect issues until the relationship was solid and the dangerous behaviour stopped.

If you speak to people who have been injured in their work with horses, you will hear about shortcuts they took (not so much a knowledge issue as a judgement issue), and you may also hear examples from the "didn't know that I didn't know" category. This is one reason you may hear Fjord owners express concern about promoting the breed as good for beginners. A well-trained, properly-cared-for Norwegian Fjord horse is probably going to be calmer, friendlier, and more forgiving than a similar horse of many other breeds. However, there are potential buyers who see a calm, cute, seemingly cuddly small horse and—if they don't make the time to learn—may not have a clue about the damage that can be done by an intelligent half-tonne warm-blooded package of muscle and bone that can compete with Clydesdales in draft sports. In an online forum I follow, a woman referred to Fjords as the Harley-Davidsons of the horse world. Such cautions apply to any breed of horse. Think about the other myths you may have heard: *draft horses are calm; ponies are great for kids;* and so on. Any romantic notions can lead to big risks. As Gayle Ecker from Equine Guelph says: "If all you want is a fuzzy bicycle, don't get a horse."

Some gaps in knowledge can be deadly, horses die because of what owners don't know they don't know. Lisa Ross Williams describes the work of Chris Pollitt, director of the Australian Equine Laminitis Research Unit at Queensland University. Pollitt says that chronic laminitis and founder are the second-biggest killers of horses after colic. Laminitis and founder are closely related (and sometimes you will hear people use the terms synonymously). Laminitis is an inflammation of the sensitive laminae, which carry blood to the parts of the hoof. It is caused by a change in the blood supply and can be excruciatingly painful for the horse (and emotionally painful for the person who has to care for the horse). In some cases the hoof wall and the coffin bone (the bone closest to the ground) come apart, and the bone sinks downward, possibly even puncturing the sole of the foot. I have only seen a horse with laminitis once, and it was heartbreaking. I couldn't imagine how painful the experience was for the horse or for his owner.

Colic is the number one killer of horses. Colic has many forms but is always associated with abdominal pain and usually results from the intestine being distended. It requires immediate treatment by a veterinarian.

	TRUE OR FALSE
1.	Morning grazing after an overnight freeze is better than after a mild night.
2.	Hay from fertilized fields is better than unfertilized.
3.	Healthy, lush, long grass is preferable to short, scrubby grass.
4.	If you mow a pasture before putting your horses out, they will get less sugar.
5.	On a sunny day, grazing in the morning is better than the afternoon.

Table 3: Grazing Quiz for Easy Keepers. Answers on p. 141

There are several causes of these conditions, but they can all relate to feed choices. When discussing easy keepers such as draft horses, Fjords, and Morgans, I have heard statements such as "grass in the morning is fine" or "grass late in the day is fine" or "long [or scrubby, short] grass is fine" or "less than *x* hours a day is fine." As you start to understand the digestive tract of your horse, and how we have changed environmental conditions for our horses, you realize it isn't that simple. Horses evolved as grazers, wandering over great distances and keeping their digestive tracts full of food. Now it is common for horses to be confined and fed two large meals per day. For a glimpse into the complexities, Table 3 is a short quiz to test your knowledge, and a list of grazing tips from Colorado State University follows. Answer the questions with True (T) or False (F), assuming you are trying to prevent a horse from having too much sugar but are allowing modest grazing periods.

Good grazing management will lower the consumption of fructan and reduce the incidence of colic and laminitis.

Fructan is a non-structural carbohydrate (NSC), like simple sugars and starches, but is different from sugar and starch because it must be fermented in the hindgut like other "fibre-type" complex carbohydrates. Fermentation of fructan, other complex carbohydrates, and fibre involves a longer process than fermentation of sugar and starch. It also requires a delicate balance of the proper population of micro-organisms in the hindgut. Good practices should include the following:

- Limit grazing on high-fructan grasses: no more than one hour per day for susceptible horses.
- Use grazing muzzles when necessary.
- Don't overgraze pastures.
- Consider fertilized fields or buying hay from fertilized fields.
- Graze early morning as the norm.
- After a sunny day and a cold night, limit grazing in the morning: the plant has not used up its energy store of fructan during the night.

Joanne Meszoly cites forage researcher Kathryn Watts, who adds another complicating factor. In order to increase weight gain and milk production in cattle, many plant breeders are deliberately increasing carbohydrate levels in new grass varieties. Some horse owners may not even realize their horses are accessing new and "improved" grass varieties. There are many nuances when it comes to sugars in grasses, so I highly recommend you learn more about the grasses in your area and about the grazing situations that could put your horse at risk. Talk with your vet and with a nutritionist as key resource people. I have not mentioned grains here, but colic can result from a horse getting into a grain supply. Make certain this doesn't happen. Many people use old, out-of-reach, and even locked freezers for storing grain

We have delved into a few examples of learning here, but there are many more. Ask any professional and you will hear about misinformation related to his or her field: how to get weight off a horse, how to set up a worming schedule, how to judge the quality of hay, and so on. For example, Ray M. Kaplan, a professor of parasitology at the University of Georgia's College of Veterinary Medicine's Department of Infectious Diseases, has seen a lot of misinformation about worming. Think about this: every case of very serious parasitic infections he has seen, which often led to deaths, was on a farm where horses were dewormed very frequently. People who learned about worming schedules a long time ago were learning about the control of bloodworms, which are very dangerous for horses but are rare now.

Learning to speak equestrian is a lifelong pursuit. Every time we encounter a new area of knowledge (tack, dressage, groundwork, probiotics, deworming schedules, hoof care, hay composition, first aid, companion animals, and so on), we have choices. Do we tune out and perhaps argue with others, thinking we know enough? Do we feel inadequate and delay the learning? Or do we open up to ways of learning so that we can access new and important information quickly when we need it? Some of you may love learning; you may already be actively involved in building skills and knowledge in other areas. Or perhaps it has been a while since you dove into a new area, and it might feel overwhelming. As a beginner myself, I want to encourage you. Despite the periodic stressors of differentiating between different opinions, it is energizing to learn, to be the best horse owner you can be, and even to periodically help others when they have questions.

POINTS TO PONDER

▶ Become a master of open-ended questions in your mission to speak equestrian.

▶ Find a coach. Find a good coach. Treasure a good coach.

▶ Learn by experience. Terms are helpful; knowing what to do with terms is powerful.

▶ Horses move beautifully without a rider, but they need to learn how to carry a rider without damaging their bodies.

▶ Realize there is a lot to learn. Don't always trust your intuition about what you need, and realize there are risks to not knowing.

▶ Each horse is different and some will test your best efforts at horse-proofing.

▶ Some well-intentioned feeding habits can be bad for your horse; they can even kill your horse.

▶ Learn about new research related to nutrition and parasites; trust the latest science for these topics that can be life-threatening for your horse.

||||||||||||||||||||||||||||||||||||||||||||||||||||||||||||||||||||||
QUESTION TO CONSIDER
||||||||||||||||||||||||||||||||||||||||||||||||||||||||||||||||||||||

▶ How will you deal with people you care about who have strong opinions that don't match those of experts such as veterinary medicine researchers? (Read on!)

Answers to Quiz on p. 138: 1) F, 2) T, 3) F, 4) F, 5) T

Our choicest plans have fallen through,
our airiest castles tumbled over,
because of lines we neatly drew
and later neatly stumbled over.

PIET HEIN "ON PROBLEMS"

11 | Learning to Make Your Own Decisions

ASK QUESTIONS and you will get opinions. Lots of them. Some opinions vary because of different contexts. For example, water management in Fairbanks will be different than in Seattle. The value of free lunging for a calm, supple horse will be different than for a high-headed, stressed, and counter-bent one. Some opinions will blatantly conflict with each other. You may find yourself in that awkward position of having good friends, relatives, or respected coaches who absolutely disagree about what you should do. In this chapter, I share some of my experiences—successful and not so successful—with decision making.

About a year after getting Bocina, I decided to take her to a natural horsemanship clinic. Natural horsemanship employs ways of working with horses based on horse body language and psychology. Many women are drawn to natural horsemanship, a philosophy that swings the pendulum away from the old extreme horse-breaking methods that were rooted in fear and control.

There are many natural horsemanship clinicians. I chose Jonathan Field, largely because people I respected from both Western and English traditions had recommended him. I had watched some of his videos and seen some of his techniques practised. Although I was looking forward to the clinic, I had reservations. I knew Bocina's previous owner had some objections to natural horsemanship approaches, as did my riding coach. I knew from some of my natural horsemanship friends that they had concerns about elements of dressage. So was I going to confuse my horse? Become confused myself? Jeopardize friendships?

I was correct in that—at least on the surface—I was being asked to do things my coach might not like. So I needed to find ways to make (and perhaps revise) decisions within some frameworks.

Finding a Framework

During the four-day clinic, we began each day by coming into the arena without our horses, doing some review, and asking questions. I asked Jonathan about the apparent contradictions we encounter from books and clinicians and friends. I told him my horse was trained in dressage, but I was obviously interested in natural horsemanship as well. He quickly sketched the first of my "frameworks." It looked something like the figure on the next page.

Jonathan described why he sees natural horsemanship and the communication and mutual respect it enables as the foundation of all disciplines. He positioned reining and dressage at the next level—for Western and English riding respectively—because of the comprehensive skills and detailed communication with your horse that these disciplines

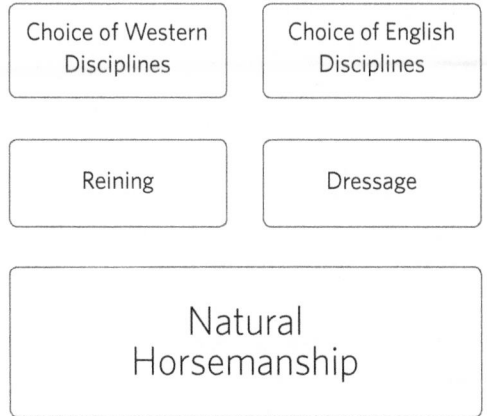

Figure 2: *Jonathan Field's sketch*

demand. With those two layers under your belt, you are well positioned to work with cutting, roping, eventing, jumping, trail riding, or whatever other activities are right for you and your horse. Not everyone would agree with this framework, but it provided lots of food for thought.

With this framework in mind, I could focus on desired outcomes more than apparent contradictions. The framework didn't make the decisions for me, but at the very least, it showed me how people like Jonathan think about these questions and find complementary relationships and natural flows of learning. This particular framework might not work for you, but I encourage you to find ways of sorting through the conflicting direction you will encounter. And always keep people's fragile egos in mind. There are many respectful ways of setting aside someone's advice, at least for the short term.

Our society encourages us to use our logical minds to make important decisions. You have probably been told "Just make two columns: one with pros and one with cons, and weigh them: the answer will be obvious." That system works well for some decisions. However, for relationship-building activities, consider another approach: 1) Keep learning about yourself and how to be authentically aware and attentive in the moment; 2) Keep learning about your horse's temperament, body language, and responsiveness; 3) Make intuitive choices in the moment; and 4) Learn from those choices by dropping what isn't working and building on what is. In *The Tao of Equus*, Linda Kahanov writes:

> I had seen training strategies that sounded perfectly reasonable in theory cause all kinds of problems in the riding arena, while impulses that seemed to make no sense at all often worked effortlessly. As my own mind formed a reciprocal relationship with feeling, instinct and intuition, my success with horses increased exponentially.

I have even heard experienced people, such as Carolyn Resnick being interviewed by Stormy May, say that great trainers have learned to become comfortable with not knowing what they are doing. In learning to make our own decisions, we need to live in that paradox. We need to use logic where logic works. And we need to be so open to observation and learning—about ourselves, our horses, and our environments—that we shed decades of protective assumptions. Part of learning is unlearning. We need to recapture a child-like world view in which magic is possible and constraints are few.

Learning the Hard Way

Fortunately, most thoughtfully made poor decisions do not have serious, long-term consequences. Here are two of the errors I have made that I still squirm about:

1. Buying a horse property (or—more accurately—buying a property on which I could keep my horse).

We could not afford the kinds of properties you see listed as horse properties, so I was looking for a small acreage where I could store some hay, have a run-in shed for my mare, and have a paddock area for her that did not interfere with things such as the septic field or groundwater quality. We looked for two years, spending countless hours on the web, driving by places for sale, and having several visits with each of two realtors. Promising listings would be pulled off the market just as we booked appointments to see them. Properties that looked good on paper had serious flaws. It was beginning to look impossible. Then we started to look on a small island, which we realized could be inconvenient. However, property values were a bit lower. We found a property smaller than we'd hoped for, and after many conversations with regulators, we determined we could have Bocina on the property. So we bought it. I had the bottom of the property (run-in shed and paddock area) cleared and had a beautiful little hay shed with a tiny tack-up area built at the top of the property. Then I carried on with the research I had started about the footing: how to ensure the paddock was dry enough, whether we had to use landscape cloth to prevent any noxious weeds from growing through, and so on.

As I did this, I started getting feedback from locals that my plans were simply not practical. Gravel and sand were very expensive on the island. And to make matters worse, the layout of the property would require people to cart vast quantities of gravel down a hill in wheelbarrows. I had spent decades saving and two years searching for the right place— and had bought the wrong place. I could not keep my horse on the property, I could not look out the window and see her from the kitchen or pull on boots over my pyjamas and take her a flake of hay in the morning. I recall the elevator-dropping feeling when I finally figured this out. This was the most expensive mistake of my life. But, it's okay. There are some upsides to the story. And Bocina is just as happy—maybe happier—living with other horses in self-board settings. Yet there is always an undercurrent of angst: What if I had to move her and there were no suitable boarding options on the island?

2. She'll be happier with a bit of grass.
   This one isn't surprising. I was one of those mothers who let my kids figure things out on their own. I have few dictatorial bones in my body: it is all about communication and consensus. This bit-of-grass problem bit us twice.

   The first time was at West Coast boarding location number one. They had a Western hitching post, which was about three feet high. I had only worked with higher crossties. Bocina had been there for a few weeks and our interactions were basic: grooming, feeding, walks, and a bit of trail riding with a coach alongside on foot.

   I had her out of her run-in shed/paddock area and tied to the hitching post for the first time and was grooming her. The section of rope attached to her halter was perhaps three feet long; she could reach down to a very small area of grass (which was a rare treat for her, as there was no fenced area in which she could graze). All of a sudden she was tangled. She had somehow stepped through the rope with her right hind leg and was panicking. I don't know that I had read the advice to put your own safety ahead of your horse's. If I had read it, I ignored it. I had learned the knot that allowed me to pull and release (but not the one that allowed *either* Bocina or me to release it). I reached over, pulled, and the crisis was averted within a few seconds. No physical damage done. You need to learn the ropes (so to speak) and learn the knots.

This lack of discipline came back to haunt us a second time about a year later at a different self-boarding facility. I had trained her not to graze on a rope without my permission, and she was usually good about that. However, one day was different. I put her saddle on, unhooked her halter, and put on her bridle. All buckles were done up except the throatlatch. I had left that buckle until last, because I was going to use side reins. I reached under her neck to twist the reins and thread the throatlatch through them, so there was no chance she could trip on her reins while being lunged. She dropped her big Fjord head and neck at lightning speed to grab a mouthful of grass, and a split second later, she stepped on the throatlatch. She jerked her head up and her bridle was ripped and tangled around her face. Again, I managed to untangle her quickly. There appeared to be no damage, though she was frightened. But she was difficult when being lunged by my coach later that day, and I eventually realized it was because her face was very sore, especially around the noseband. And a few months later when her teeth were being floated, the vet noted a tooth scar on her tongue, which may have been part of that mishap. A kind intent can become a cruel reality.

Nothing horrific resulted from these poor decisions. But they give hints of what can happen when someone does not learn from mistakes. Perhaps you have seen or heard of horses who lose respect for humans and become dangerous, not because they are "bad" horses, but because people have avoided discipline in order to be kind, or liked, or for some other motive, which is probably connected with unresolved issues in their own lives. A healthy relationship is about a healthy, empowered you, your trusting horse, and the space of respect and possibility in between.

Day-to-Day Decisions

As you work with your horse over time, you will be learning about nutrition, first aid, barn management, tack, training, and more. Earlier, I described the basic preparation I did for my horse's arrival: buying food, bedding, tack, and the like. Here, I describe a few of the additions or changes I made over the following twelve months. They fit into the category of somewhat mundane day-to-day decision-making processes, but perhaps these examples will prompt you to think about the kinds of changes you want to consider in your context.

Nutrition: At first, I matched Bocina's feed as perfectly as I could to what she was used to. This was first cut hay, a pelleted food supplement and micro-cut flax, which does not go rancid as quickly as flax milled with other methods. Later, I switched her feed for several reasons. She was being worked less and needed fewer calories; she was now in an environment with very low selenium in the soil and hay; and I had learned more about how common GMO flax is. Based on research online and through Fjord owning friends I a) reduced her hay consumption slightly and sometimes soaked it to lower sugar content; b) shifted pellets to a locally produced product that was high selenium, low calorie and fed in smaller quantities; c) added a small amount of soaked "Fibremax" (largely soy) pellets that are low glycemic; and d) milled my own certified organic, non-GMO flax. She did well on the new regime, and I had no plans to change it in the short term. However, I was becoming increasingly aware of how much there is to learn about optimal nutrition. The next time I bought hay, I had it tested and found it was too high in carbohydrates and much too low in protein to be ideal. So that led to more short-term changes, guided by a very knowledgeable local nutritionist, Ken Wilkinson. Be curious and open to learning about nutrition for your horse's breed, age, level of activity, and environment. And always make transitions gradually.

Bridle and Bit: Although horses move beautifully in the field without training, they have to adjust the way they carry themselves with a rider. Their weight tends to be too far forward, their backs hollow, their heads too far out front and their hind legs too far back. If they stay off balance while being ridden, there can be many problems for the horse, including back pain. Many people ride without understanding these issues.

I had a lot of difficulty getting Bocina to make good contact with the bit, get her back rounded, and get well balanced on all four legs, even though she was quite capable of doing this with a good rider. Her trot was like riding an industrial sewing machine. My neck and upper back would knot up after holding up what felt like a hundred pounds of neck. In addition to improving my riding technique, there were three interventions my coach tried to remedy this situation.

The first was draw reins. These extra woven cotton reins were an interim measure used to lower the horse's head, round her back, and get her into a position similar to the one an excellent rider would expect. This intervention is controversial, though, and I only did this for a short time under the guidance of my coach.

The second was side reins. I bought leather ones with doughnut links for some give. These have the same purpose but for lunging rather than riding. They help the horse practise a good position and presumably feel as though she has a skilled rider holding the reins. But we still weren't getting great results.

The third intervention was a Pelham bit with adaptors for single reins. This is a more controlling bit in case that is needed. Some people were concerned about this choice, but Bocina did not object to the bit, and it enabled me to get the "feel" of a properly connected horse and a really nicely measured trot. I was then able to transfer that back to the snaffle without using draw reins.

The bridle and bit are key pieces of tack for communication. They can relay your intentions and reassure a horse. They can also confuse, irritate, or hurt a horse. Make decisions carefully and remember that your skills and the tack truly work hand in hand with these items.

Horse Boots: A general rule is to keep and ride your horse on similar footings. For example, if your horse lives in a field with soft dirt and grass, she may find it uncomfortable to ride on a gravel road or creek bed. In her previous home, my horse was ridden in a sand arena. Now her pastures are dirt (AKA mud in the winter), and we are not often in a ring. She has never been shod, and I would prefer to keep it that way. So when we go out on dirt trails she is fine, but on gravel road hills or creek bed trails, her feet are sometimes sensitive. So I added boots (in our case, Cavallo simple boots for front hooves) to her wardrobe, and so far they are working fine. Some people suggest I get gators to insert in the boots to prevent rubbing, but so far the soft edges of the boots have prevented any problems.

Girth: I bought a leather dressage girth, which was essentially identical to the one she was used to. But now she was starting to spend more time on slopes. On one ride, the dressage girth rubbed and there was a small sore behind her leg. Several of the women who own horses on the island chipped in for a major birthday of mine and gave me a beautiful girth with a removable sheepskin covering. This works very well for trail rides on cool days.

Safety Vest: At good tack shops, you will see vests designed to protect a rider if she falls. The comfortable ones are not cheap. At one point my coach suggested I get one; at the time Bocina was nervous about the dark forests, narrow trails and occasional unpredictable wildlife sightings along them. So I got a vest and felt rejuvenated when the store owner gave me the discount a new, young rider would get through 4H membership. I don't wear it all the time, but it is reassuring to have it for certain circumstances. The vest purchase also reminded me to wear a helmet for groundwork. Many people don't do this, but I have heard stories of serious injuries from events as innocuous as a horse swinging his head around to bite a fly.

Science, Friendly Advice, and Folklore

Lastly, a few comments on the kinds of information you will encounter. Scientific information is likely to come from sources such as your vet and websites for extension services of veterinary colleges. This information will typically be based on well-conducted studies using scientific methods. Value this information highly, but be aware it may be out of date or based on work with a breed very different from yours, or it may ignore wisdom from other ways of knowing.

Friendly advice is not necessarily less valid or less valuable than scientific information. For example, if you need help with some issue and post (perhaps with photos to help people understand) on a big online forum, you might get a dozen responses reflecting many decades of practical experience, including ideas or details not covered in the scientific literature. Don't rush. Allan Hamilton writes: "Whenever an impasse is reached with a horse, stop. Ask yourself: How would I approach this problem if I were given a hundred years to solve it?"

Folklore may seem the least valuable source of information, but don't write it off. Consider an Iranian Arab breeder's interpretation of the Bedouin notion that a horse with a right front white sock is bad luck. In a culture where science is glorified we tend to roll our eyes at statements about "bad luck." But Linda Tellington-Jones shares insights about this mythology. Bedouin warriors carried their weapons over their right shoulders. This would put more weight over the white-socked hoof, and dark hooves are stronger than white ones. Folklore and science may be coming together here to explain why Bedouins wisely made certain choices.

POINTS TO PONDER

- ▶ Be prepared to hear very different opinions, about almost everything, from experienced people.
- ▶ Pay attention to inconsistencies in advice. They are opportunities for gathering information and for learning about yourself.
- ▶ Try to find or develop some sort of a framework so that you can put different opinions in context and make sense of them.
- ▶ Pay close attention to what is happening in the moment with your horse and build on successes.
- ▶ Realize you will make mistakes.
- ▶ List three criteria to guide your decisions about changes, purchases, or how you treat your horse. Put them on your fridge door or the wall of the barn or both.
- ▶ Make changes to diet thoughtfully and gradually.
- ▶ As you learn, think about all this new knowledge as a sort of buffet. The buffet includes your own experiences with your horse, science, ideas from experienced horse owners, books, and other sources. As

you try to make progress or work through a challenge, take one or two items from the buffet and try them out. Pay close attention to how they work, learn, and repeat.

QUESTION TO CONSIDER

▸ Think about my bit-of-grass story that revealed one of my weak-nesses. What are yours? What are your strengths? (Strengths and weaknesses can sometimes be the same.) How will they improve or compromise your decisions?

||||||||||||||||||||

Calvin: You know, Hobbes,
some days even my lucky rocket ship
underpants don't help.

BILL WATTERSON

12 | Fear and Courage

A SKILLED HORSEWOMAN who read drafts of
this book asked, "Are you going to have a chapter on fear?"
She was referring to fear in humans, not horses. The more I
thought about that, the more important it seemed. Yet by its
very nature, it's a difficult topic to address. Let me begin by
telling a story that isn't about horses but affects my relationship with my horse.

In my early fifties I decided I *definitely* wasn't going to get
a PhD. I had saved a small amount of money towards tuition
and found it was enough to get a second-hand motorbike. I
had a demanding career, which I had often juggled with university courses. I deserved a treat. This was going to be easy
and fun. At the time, I regularly cycled to work, so my balance
and strength were pretty good. I had driven standard cars, so
understood the basics of transmissions and gears. And I had
ridden as a passenger on motorbikes in my twenties.

I signed up for lessons at a reputable school. The courses were intense, spanning many hours per day over several days. It was the fall (great temperatures for riding), and I was catching the second-last set of lessons in the year. After some orientation and introductory material, they gave each of us a 250cc motorbike and we headed out to the parking lot, bordered on one side by a steep man-made hill. The instructor went over how the throttle, clutch, gears, and brakes worked. There are scientific studies that say most women have more trouble with spatial things than men do. I was experiencing that in spades. Standing there with the bike, I just could not envision how all these things fit together and what I should do to move ahead and stop. Others started pulling out, riding at slow speed around the parking lot. The ex-military instructor was increasingly impatient with me. Eventually, he more or less ordered me to get into the line. I did, and all went well for a few seconds. Then I was heading up that extremely steep embankment, terrified I was going to go over the top. Fortunately, I fell, with the bike on top of me. I never mentioned that I chipped my shinbone. I got back on and eventually figured it out but was really shaken. Because this slowed my progress, I had to stay into the evening to catch up. As I was doing slow manoeuvres (which are difficult on a motorbike) around cones, I fell again, this time spraining my fingers. Off to the hospital I went, had my wedding ring cut off, went back home, and rebooked lessons for the final set.

Yes, I "got back on the bike." And I bought a beautiful bike. There were times when getting through that learning curve and riding a motorbike made me a stronger woman. I dealt with breast cancer not long after the bike lessons. After the surgery, each weekday morning I would dress up in protective black leather chaps and jacket, ride to the hospital for the first available radiation appointment of the day, ride to work (only ten minutes late), and walk into the building still in black leathers. I think it is one of the reasons I beat cancer, taking only eight days of vacation off work.

Yet I never shook the fear from that first day of lessons. I was always an extremely cautious rider. I almost never went on trips longer than city errands and commuting. I never went out with other riders, feeling somehow inferior or less skilled. I never took on a passenger. And although there were moments when I felt absolute joy, they merely punctuated the underlying angst that I never managed to shed.

The fearless child seems to be a common theme when mature women talk about their revised attitudes towards horses. I recall when I finally got permission to ride Joe after watching him through the fence for years. I was probably fourteen. I had never seen him ridden. I didn't know what breed he was or anything about how he behaved under saddle. But when I got the okay, I was absolutely thrilled. I had no fear whatsoever. On July 1 (Canada's birthday), I went out for a ride and he bucked me off (I thought it was because of a horsefly bite, and it may have been). To me, this was exciting, a great story about my Canada Day adventure. I was glad I had a helmet on and relieved I wasn't hurt, but I had no misgivings about getting back on. I hear similar (and much wilder) horse stories about women in their youth. But I have not yet met one who has retained all of that fearlessness.

I mentioned my broken shoulder in chapter 1. Right after the injury, when I got to a phone, I called my husband rather than 911 because a call from a paramedic would worry him more. He said something like "It was bound to happen." He considered injury an inevitable part of work with a horse. Certainly, when I was injured, it opened the door for lots of stories from others about their injuries. But these tales of injuries were told as unfortunate accidents in otherwise very satisfying lives. They were often told with humour. Many stories were duets of sorts: the memories of central characters and witnesses woven together like pieces of theatre. This was shared history, part of the fabric of learning, relationship building, survival, and celebration that happens between human and equine friends. If we had an injury-free human-horse decade, we would forget how powerful these magnificent animals are and how we need to interact in specific ways, ways that are different than life with a dog, cat, or child.

When the topic of accidents comes up, horse people seem to want to know details, perhaps in the hope that they will glimpse some pattern or lesson to drop into their pool of knowledge, thereby avoiding similar injuries to themselves or relatives or friends. The insight I gain from a story might be different than the one you gain, or that your friend gains. So in that spirit, I will share the details of my story.

I broke my shoulder in a horse accident that truly was an accident. It might have been preventable, but one could say that about every accident, whether it be in a car or on a ski slope.

It was a cool, damp November day. My horse was in her usual fenced field: a long, narrow forested field, close to an acre in size, at the back of the property where I have the self-board arrangement. She was the only horse in the field, though she could easily see the other mare—Cara—in a parallel field with a long, skinny paddock between them. Cara is a Thoroughbred, much more skittish than Bocina, and has always become easily herd-bound. Bocina is usually the dominant mare, and Cara watches her closely. If Bocina goes out of sight, Cara panics until she is visible again.

To ride Bocina off the property, I needed to get both horses down through fields—including slippery, muddy sections—to the barn. Cara may get upset in a stall, but she is unlikely to hurt herself. When Cara first arrived on the property, it felt a bit like those children's math puzzles where you read about having a canoe, a cabbage, a sheep, and a wolf, and you have to get them all across the river in *x* trips without anything being eaten.

At the time of the accident, the safest way to move them was with two people, one with each horse. On this day, I was alone and didn't have a lot of time. So I decided to work with Bocina in the field. This was somewhat unfamiliar to her: the field was—in a sense—her home without rules, in contrast to work in a ring or on trails, where expectations were more firmly established.

The only tack I took into the field was a rope halter with a twelve-foot lead rope, which can also be used for reins. We did a few activities in the field, moving hindquarters and shoulders in both directions, backing up, flexing the neck, and so on. There was a sort of mounting block, and I decided to ride a bit bareback, which we rarely do. If using the rope halter and reins, one should really do a large complex knot under the halter to decrease the length of the reins. But this was only going to be a very brief ride, and I was having trouble with the knot. So I did a simpler knot and left the reins long. When I mounted, I wasn't quite centred. She kept walking and wouldn't whoa, so I slipped off her back to eliminate the discomfort. She seemed calm, but these unfamiliar activities probably had her a bit more energized than usual.

There is a well-worn path along the edge of the field from when Cara lived in the field and paced the fence line. We were walking along this fence line towards the lower fields and barn, with me on the left, then Bocina, then the fence, then the skinny paddock and the other field with Cara to my far right. My memory is a bit vague, but I think the rope reins slipped down and Bocina stepped through with her right foreleg. She didn't seem at all concerned. I reached over in front of her. I could not have been more than four feet in front of her chest and probably much less. A second later, she hit me with unbelievable force. I went up in the air and landed on my left shoulder, or left arm and shoulder.

She stopped as quickly as she started. I knew I was injured, though I didn't guess about details. As I hit, I had three thoughts in rapid succession. 1) This is serious. 2) My friend Jane (who re-assessed life priorities and reconnected with horses after she had part of her arm amputated) can do everything with one arm; this shouldn't cause too many problems. And 3) Bocina has stopped and has no intention of moving. I don't need to worry about her walking or running over me.

Then I felt a soft, warm muzzle on the back of my neck, and she kept nuzzling me until I was able to get up. I used my right hand to undo the rope halter and dragged the gear as I walked down the field very slowly. When we practice working together on the ground with no tack (liberty work), I am lucky to have her walk with me without tack for more than thirty feet. But she stayed right with me, matching my extremely slow pace, all the way down the field. Of course the next field (I had to just open the gate and let her through) had grass, and I was no competition for that.

I got to a phone, and eventually to a hospital. Apparently I was in the emergency department for about twenty-four hours, but I don't remember that. When I was moved to a ward, I had great nurses on what they assured me was the best floor of the hospital. My shoulder was a bit of a mess.

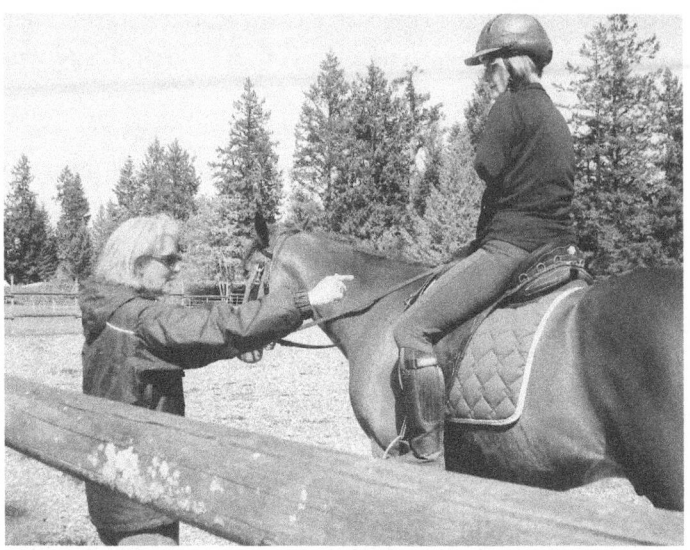

ABOVE *Coach Deborah Fox gives Jane some tips. Deborah and Jane have worked with Donny, an assertive off-track Standardbred, to help him be a safe, responsive trail companion for Jane.* Photo: ALICE MACGILLIVRAY

Things were pushed into positions they shouldn't be in. There were fractures through the top and down the outer edge of the humerus. Part of a bone was crushed. It took thirty hours to get me into surgery. Ironically, this was— in part—because of the number of surgeries in the queue related to serious dog injuries.

Two weeks later, the surgeon sent me for an emergency CT scan, which confirmed that all the rotator cuff muscles had come loose, so a second surgery was required. That was the most difficult part. I felt poisoned from all the drugs, and the second surgery was much more painful. However, the engineers who designed the hardware used in the first operation had been very thoughtful and provided holes in a plate that enabled the surgeon to easily reattach the muscles. Thank you, engineers, wherever you are. Could I buy you a beer?

When I returned home, I watched far too many black-and-white classic movies from the sofa. It was a slow recovery but moved along at a reasonable pace. At my age, I wondered if my bone health was good enough, despite taking what I believe are the best nutritional supplements available. Tests showed my bones are great; the breaks were simply from the type and force of impact.

I did not experience fear when I was injured or during the recovery process. Despite this, I want to emphasize the significance of what can happen when you are careless, have not maintained training properly, misread horse body language, or are just plain unlucky. Think about it. My calm-natured, well-trained horse moved approximately three feet from standing still and caused multiple breaks and crushed bone in a woman who is healthy and has good bone strength. These animals are incredibly powerful. And they are animals, flight-oriented prey animals at that, with their own rules about behaviour with each other that we beginners have not learned. They are horses, not dogs. Who knows if they love us (whatever that really means), but they clearly don't love us in exactly the same way a woman loves a horse. Don't fall into the disturbingly common trap of thinking, "My horse loves me; he would never hurt me." Don't confuse boundaries with being unkind. Don't confuse growing trust with immunity. And don't confuse courage with a mastery of horse behaviour. Klaus Pfungst narrates a video in which a woman is injured by her horse as they run around a paddock "playing." When you learn to speak even a little bit of horse, you see the horse is upset by the "play," and not enjoying it as the woman seems to believe. Pfungst suggests she might not have even learned the lesson of misinterpretation through the experience of being injured.

As I started to work with Bocina again, some of the feelings I had as a result of learning to ride a motorbike came back. I was anxious, mostly around my lack of confidence. Would I know—for example—if she was moving into my space more than she should? And if so, did I have the skills to correct it properly and quickly? What if I accidentally took a rope in my left hand and she jerked it, when I was not supposed to work that arm at all? And so on.

In the spring, I was allowed to ride again (with a Pelham bit). I remember the first day I tacked her up to ride her off the property, which can be a sticky spot. She had been acting up a little bit for my friend Bonnie during their rides together. I was slightly nervous, and knew I could not hide that from Bocina. My way of dealing with it was the same way I dealt with that day of being "in my head" that I talked about in chapter 8. I went up to her face and really focused on trying to communicate. Although she only knows a few words of English (and her coach swears she can spell "trot"), I used words as well as images. I said something like "I *am* a bit anxious but not afraid. If you could just take care of me today, it would be so good." I don't know what she understood, but I know she was listening. And she behaved beautifully. No hesitations. And she even walked smartly up the first hill where she often labours as though she were on the last stretch of some Nepalese mountain.

Geraldine is a local horsewoman who wrestles with fear. Her daughter was keen on riding, so they found a horse property and bought two horses. However, these relatively calm horses didn't match her daughter's dream of what Geraldine referred to as "hot-blooded psycho beauties." So the parents inherited the horses. "I had no horse experience," Geraldine told me, and there were all sorts of surprises: "Romeo was used to being out on pasture with a herd; he had never had grain. So we put some in a little bowl and he got super excited and territorial and turned around and bucked and I thought: we've bought a horse from hell."

In fact, they quickly learned that he was a very calm horse. "You could throw a big ball at him, and he'd say: 'that's nice; can you eat it?'" But the bucking incident stuck in her mind. Geraldine usually rides Venus, a 14.3-hand mare. They get along beautifully on the ground. "She'll walk or run along beside me without a lead rope; it's an amazing feeling," says Geraldine. But riding isn't going so well. "Sometimes my legs shake so badly, I dismount. I'm a nervous wreck, and I make her a nervous wreck. It must be like having a cougar on her back. I can't canter; I'm not comfortable trotting; I've fallen a few times and that really sets me back."

I asked her why she has hung in there, given all the learning, the expenses, her daughter's not taking to the horses, and the fear. She can't imagine giving up an animal she has taken on, and she feels very close to Venus. But the fear obstacle is in the way. "I've even tried drinking," she said, and I laughed, thinking she was joking. But it was one of several techniques she has seriously tried. "I don't drink, but I thought I really need something to calm me down." That wasn't the solution, but she has found a good mentor/coach and is constantly working to develop the skills and confidence she wants to have. Her successful solutions will come, and they might be quite different than the next person's.

We've all met people who thrive in situations most of us would find terrifying. Hormones, experience, and other factors play into whether we feel fear and how we react to it. It makes sense to have a healthy respect for horses and to be afraid when we're at risk of injury. Fear exists to help us survive. Yet, as Geraldine described, fear can circle from human to horse and back in a feedback loop of emotion and energy. But think back to some of the successes in your life that never would have happened without overcoming fear. Perhaps taking a leap in your career, learning to ride a bicycle, opening up to friendships, moving to a new place, getting married, becoming a mother. Without reasonable doses of fear, life would be safe but not rewarding. The art is in learning how to make a habit of courage.

Phil Odden recently asked me if I had ever considered the concept that the horse will eventually take on the personality of the handler. That got me thinking of a whole other cycle of courage and fear. If I don't build the confidence I need to be the kind of horsewoman Phil would truly respect, then I am not only compromising the relationship with my horse. I am also compromising the potential of my horse.

This chapter represents my immediate experience, and through conversations with many experts I have come to realize my experience is somewhat naive. Everyone can experience fear and courage. For some, the fear and courage are grounded in knowledge, experience, and respect. Without respect and knowledge, courage is dangerous.

POINTS TO PONDER

▶ Make a list of strengths or assets you have already, from any aspect of your life, to have a healthily fearless relationship with your horse.

▶ Periodically test your knowledge of horse body language by observing with a knowledgeable friend, or by watching narrated videos on the web or from clinicians with the sound turned off for the first viewing.

QUESTION TO CONSIDER

▸ If you became afraid of some aspect of work with your horse, what
ten approaches might help you work constructively through that
fear?

A man on a horse is spiritually
 as well as physically
bigger than a man on foot.

JOHN STEINBECK

13 | Where Might This Road Take You?

SOME HORSEWOMEN HAVE commented that, as they age, they shift the nature of their activities with horses. Many talk about wanting quiet relationships: perhaps walking on trails when they used to compete. Many also talk about spending more time on the ground with their horses. For example, a friend often goes out late in the evening, sometimes by moonlight, and gives her horses long grooming sessions, which they love. A few have told me they switched from riding most of the time to driving more often, as it was easier on the body. And a few have become competitive, when they didn't really think that shows or competitions were of interest to them. I have mentioned that Fjords are known for their versatility. Of course that usually means they can do almost everything, but they are not likely to be competing at the highest levels in anything. But there are some exceptions. Fjords with skilled trainers often do very well with driving competitions. Phil Odden had competed

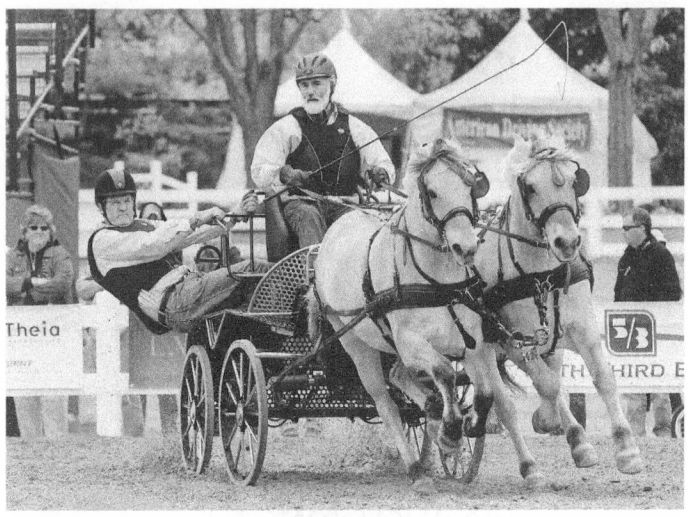

ABOVE *Phillip Odden driving Silver Willow Marcy and Ke Ja Co's Herger at the 2010 Alltech FEI World Equestrian Games. Howard Fiedler is leaning into the turn as navigator.* Photo: ELSE BIGTON

successfully with his Fjords in many competitions, often placing well above other breeds.

What would we lose if we no longer had horses and our relationships with horses? After all, horses aren't as essential as they were a century ago, and they can be a luxury in a tough economy. Fifty women from my online communities shared with me their views of such a loss.

The women's responses suggest that once horses are part of your life, there may be no turning back. Corinne Logan said that she will always have a horse, because she missed so much in her young adult years when she did not have horses. One woman made light of a very common theme by writing: "I always say—horses are a lot cheaper than therapy!" And another shared that "they are my family now. My husband of 45 years has passed on and I'd lose everything that I live for." And I love Bonnie's question about whether she "looked twenty" to drivers who passed her on the road:

> I was crazy for horses when I was young, and rode quite a bit during my late teens and early twenties. I attended a year-round Western riding camp where there were lots of wonderful trails, and we had a ring to ride in as well. I met a couple of horsemen who gave me some good lessons, and horses brought me a lot of goodness during those years. Over the next 30+ years I rode when I had the chance, but never enough to reestablish that warm connection and confidence that I remember from those young years.
>
> When I moved to the West Coast, I never imagined horses as part of the picture. And then, because of Alice's accident, I began to ride and care for Bocina. I rode her on trails and eventually began taking dressage lessons, feeling quite dapper on that English saddle in my helmet and half-chaps. And one day I was riding along the road after a very satisfying ride in the woods and I began to think about how familiar it all felt, and how I felt like a twenty year old up on that little Fjord mare. And a car passed and I wondered if I looked twenty to them, my sixty years all hidden under my helmet. Because I felt just like that horse-crazy young woman again.

I live on an island where many people are interested in living more sustainably. Most of us have spent time in cities and understand the benefits and costs of doing so. We only have about 4500 full time residents, but the accomplishments are extraordinary. There is a communally governed commons, a medical centre built by volunteers, "People for a Healthy Community" with creative strategies for social justice, a grain co-op, wood co-op, communal gardens, energy initiatives, and a publishing house focusing on sustainability. And this is just a sampling of initiatives. One idea I am starting to think about is to develop my skills and Bocina's so that we could help people with practical work on the land. Rather than bringing a machine to a property on a truck, perhaps Bocina and I could move sections of fallen trees? This may or may not be practical, but it is interesting to explore options.

When I asked women about what we would lose if horses were gone from our lives, I found their comments moving. Many of them used words such as therapy, sanity, activity, time outdoors, joy, happiness, wonder, learning, empowerment, warmth, beauty, teamwork and partner. However, the most common phrase surprised me: "connection with nature." These women lived in many parts of the world, in different landscapes and economies and cultures, but their relationships with their horses were tied to relationships with the natural world. There are many people in many professions trying to rekindle such relationships as we become busier, more urban, and less sensitive to the fragility of our natural environments. We now even have the phrase "nature deficit disorder," coined by Richard Louv to describe the effects on children of growing up in cities where they spend more time with electronic media and almost no time connecting with nature. Yet I have never heard any activists for sustainability say: "Spend time with horses."

A Final Thought

In this book, I have emphasized the relationships that women—particularly mature women—choose to develop with horses. And there are many reasons to do this when you see that we have become typical horse owners.

Yet I have also quoted men who care deeply about their relationships with horses. As I have spoken with women and reflected on my own experiences, I have wondered what the absence of men is really all about. In *The Path of the Horse*, or *Sur la Voie du Cheval*, independent filmmaker Stormy May shares a key learning in her work at liberty with horses (working without tack where the horse is free to express himself): "I began to see the prison I had created around myself, needing to control the circumstances in my life in order to feel safe." This sentiment resonates in so many workplace conversations and in conversations about the constraints and weights that come with masculinity in our society. Men are expected to be in control—or to give that appearance. Our heroic leader models suggest strong men should make their followers feel safe. But as a hero figure, how do you tap into the expertise of all employees? How do you effectively share leadership? How can you be masculine and kind and gentle?

Would men really rather be on the motorcycle than the horse? Ownership statistics say they would. Are women empathetic in a wider range of situations than men? Papers by Linda Rueckert, Nicolette Naybar, and others suggest so. Horseman Phil Odden notes some of the appeals of motors. They require less subtle communication skill and if they don't work you can just hand them off to someone to fix. But gender differences can be subtle, controversial, or misleading. Perhaps our culture pushes men away from discovering and enjoying equine relationships that would nourish their souls at least as much as they nourish women's. In *The Revolution in Horsemanship: And What It Means to Mankind*, Robert Miller and Richard Lamb provide us with a glimpse of male perspectives. They say that "no one becomes involved with horses to make himself a better human being or to find greater meaning in life or to make the world a better place." (Some of the women I have interviewed would take issue with that comment.) The authors go on to say: "But sometimes that's exactly what happens." Miller and Lamb offer advice such as setting your ego on the shelf while you reinvent yourself, making a commitment to act justly, and cultivating patience. They suggest the world could be a better place with benevolent leadership. And the world could also be a better place if we all became better listeners. Phil Odden said to me that with horses the fix takes time, and sometimes a horse may never be "fixed." You might move ahead, or you might even slide backwards. That is the way it always is.

I know many women (and I am among them) whose husbands have nothing to do with their horses. Many of the women are happy with that separation, but perhaps it is one that deserves more investigation. In a horse forum, one person cautioned that he has seen several relationships end when women get horses. He didn't know if this was a widespread pattern, but he found it to be an interesting observation. Others stepped in, sharing personal stories and stories from clinicians about couples separating. Perhaps horses could be a catalyst for personal development and growth of couple's relationships as well as understanding across species.

As you embark on horse ownership as a mature woman—by definition—you want *something more*. At first you may think of the "more" in simple terms, such as companionship or a partner for health and longevity. But if you really open yourself to learning, you will be in awe of the depth and breadth of feelings and interests that open up to you and your equine partner.

POINTS TO PONDER

- ► Horses open possibilities for deeper connections with nature.
- ► Relationships with horses take many forms but can be deep, powerful, and long-term and have helped many women through periods of tragedy.
- ► It seems that many men are not interested in horses or have different motivations for a relationship with a horse. But we don't really understand the differences between men and women, and they may not be as significant as they seem in the horse world.
- ► If you are in a relationship with a man, make time to explore how each of you fits into the new human-horse dynamic.

QUESTION TO CONSIDER

- ► If you have a male partner, how would you like to include him in the reawakening of your dream?

Afterword

IF THERE ARE THREE key principles I want to share, they are to be prepared, be responsible, and to become a lifelong learner in your work with horses.

Be prepared by reading and talking with people, but even more importantly, be prepared through the experiential learning you get by easing your way into horse ownership gradually.

Be responsible by knowing and respecting yourself, and respecting the living being you are welcoming into your life. If you are bringing the long-term dreams of childhood into this relationship, don't abandon the little girl's dream, but don't let the little girl make decisions that require your hard-won maturity.

Keep learning in whatever ways you can. There are important facts to learn and many good resources to help you learn them. And, at least for beginners, there are many complexities and ambiguities. When I read books by horse experts in which they sound confident with their advice, I sometimes wonder if they project confidence in order to reassure the reader who wants to learn. Or are they confident in their current stage of learning but may rethink their conclusions in the future. Or have they really figured it all out? If you find the ambiguities worrisome, just work through them as best you can and you will gain confidence about knowing and about living in the moment without knowing everything in advance.

I also find that the not knowing becomes quite fascinating. It is a bit like living a good mystery novel. Let me illustrate what I mean through two stories about haltering a horse: one about Tarot, the big Oldenburg mare you met in chapter 9, and the other about the rescued Fjord gelding, Lars, you met in chapter 3. Each owner told me a story of the horse not wanting to be haltered. You heard about how Tarot doesn't step up to the halter when Alex is looking for a horse to go trail riding—and how Alex patiently waits for the day when Tarot is ready to rediscover her love of the trails. In Lars's case, he also resisted being haltered, but Ellen's reaction was very different. In a forum post she wrote:

> This morning he was sooo funny. He thought that since he's feeling better now and we seem to be very nice to him, he would just check out how far he could go with being rude.
>
> I had offered the halter for him to stick his head in and be walked to the next pasture. He walked right past me, didn't stop when I said whoa and tried to evade the halter again. Bad boy!!!
>
> And no, he did not get away with it. The next 15 minutes he was walked, trotted, whoa-ed, put the halter on and off, backed up and circled around me until he was

smacking his lips and got the message. An hour later I came to his pasture, called him and he came to me and stuck his nose in the halter. Good boy.

Definitely trainable and like you said: also smart and a mind of his own.

Here are two very experienced horsewomen dealing with two horses, each with some baggage from previous owners. Both horses refused halters and the owners reacted very differently. Yet my intuition says they were both right. It's reminiscent of the times when a child doesn't eat dinner: do you push the child to eat or take the plate away? But here we are dealing with a thousand-pound being who speaks a different language and is trying to communicate something important: pain, anxiety, lack of focus, or a test of leadership.

As a beginner, I'd say assume there is a test of leadership; horses do that all the time. But leave your mind open for more advanced lessons down the road.

The journey is fascinating. I hope you find your paths to success and enjoy the journey even half as much as I do.

|||||||||||||||||||

References

Barry, Ellen. "Dressage vs Western, Horses." Accessed March 15, 2013, http://bit.ly/aLL6oR.

Bolender, Mark. Mountain Trail and Extreme Trail Course. *Bolender Horse Park.* Accessed March 15, 2013, http://www.bolender-horsepark.com/.

Hamilton, Allan. *Zen Mind, Zen Horse: The Science and Spirituality of Working with Horses.* North Adams, MA: Storey Publishing, 2011.

Haraway, Donna. *When Species Meet.* Minneapolis, MN: University of Minnesota Press, 2008.

Hempfling, Klaus. Hempfling Explaining Horse Accident. Accessed October 2013, http://youtu.be/MnW6RHFBfiQ

Herdy, Amy. "First Horse At 55: How One Woman Learned a Lot the Hard Way," *My Horse Daily* (blog). Accessed February 10, 2013, http://myhorse.com/blogs/english-and-western-riding/rider-education/a-first-horse-after-50-how-one-woman-learned-a-lot-the-hard-way/.

Joseph, Jenny. "When I am Old." Accessed January 2012, http://www.barbados.org/poetry/wheniam.htm.

Kaplan, Ray. *Equine Deworming Update.* Interview podcast, 1:04:32, 2013, http://www.thehorse.com/ask-the-vet/32467/equine-deworming-update.

Kohanov, Linda. *The Tao of Equus: A Woman's Journey of Healing and Transformation through the Way of the Horse.* Novato, CA: New World Library, 2001.

Lieberman, Bobbie, Linda Tellington-Jones, John Lyons, and Susan Harding. *The Ultimate Horse Behavior and Training Book.* North Pomfret, VT: Trafalgar Square Publishers, 2006.

Louv, Richard. *Last Child in the Woods: Saving our Children from Nature Deficit Disorder.* Chapel Hill, NC: Algonquin Books, 2008.

MacLeay, Jennifer. *Smart Horse: Understanding the Science of Natural Horsemanship.* Lexington, KY: Blood-Horse Publications, 2003.

Maxwell, Daniel. "Classical Horsemanship: A Phenomenological and Dramatist Study." PhD dissertation, Fielding Graduate University, 2013.

May, Stormy. *Sur la Voie du Cheval.* Accessed November, 2012, www.youtube.com/watch?v=soowHvHwTQk&feature=endscreen &NR=1.

Meszoly, Joanne. "Danger in Your Horse's Grass: Fructan." *Equisearch.* Accessed March 13, 2013, http://www.equisearch.com/horses_care/nutrition/feeds/fructandanger_032205/.

Miller, Robert, and Rick Lamb. *The Revolution in Horsemanship: And What it Means to Mankind.* Guilford, CT: Lyons Press, 2005.

Morris, Desmond. *The Naked Ape: A Zoologist's Study of the Human Animal.* London: Jonathan Cape Publishers, 1967.

Pfungst, Oskar. *Clever Hans (The Horse of Mr. Von Osten): A Contribution to Experimental Animal and Human Psychology.* Gutenberg EBook, 2010. http://www.gutenberg.org/ebooks/33936.

Rueckert, Linda, and Nicolette Naybar. "Gender Differences in Empathy: The Role of the Right Hemisphere." *Brain and Cognition* 67, Issue 2, (2008): 162–167.

Savoie, Jane. *Jane Savoie's Dressage 101: The Ultimate Source of Dressage Basics in a Language You Can Understand.* North Pomfret, VT: Trafalgar Square Books, 2011.

Scott, Naomi. *Special Needs, Special Horses: A Guide to the Benefits of Therapeutic Riding.* College Station, TX: University of North Texas Press, 2005.

Segal, Jeanne, and Melina Smith. "Emotional Intelligence: Five Key Skills for Raising Emotional Intelligence." http://www.

helpguide.org/mental/eq5_raising_emotional_intelligence.htm. Last updated March 2013.

Sheldrake, Rupert. "Rupert Sheldrake: Biologist and Author." Accessed July 3, 2012, www.rupertsheldrake.org.

Stone, Sherril. "Human Facial Discrimination in Horses: Can They Tell us Apart?" *Anim Cogn* 13:51–61. doi: 10.1007/s10071-009-0244-x (2010).

Striegel, N. "Sugar Content in Feed and Forage Affects Horses Health." *Colorado State University Extension*. Last modified October 2008, http://www.ext.colostate.edu/pubs/livestk/01818.html.

Stutz, Birgit. "Is Round Penning Beneficial to Your Horse?" *Saddle Up*, March 2013.

Tellington-Jones, Linda, and Rebecca Didier. *Dressage with Mind, Body and Soul: A 21st Century Approach to the Science and Spirituality of Riding and Horse and Rider Well-Being*. North Pomfret, VT: Trafalgar Square Publishers, 2012.

Tellington-Jones, Linda, and Sybil Taylor. *Getting in Touch with Your Horse*. North Pomfret, VT: Trafalgar Square Publishers, 2009.

University of Kentucky College of Agriculture, Food, and Environment. "Study Examines Off-The-Track Thoroughbred Adoption Issues." *The Horse: Your Guide to Equine Health Care*. http://www.thehorse.com/articles/31386/study-examines-off-the-track-Thoroughbred-adoption-issues?utm_source=Newsletter&utm_medium=bluegrass-equine-digest&utm_campaign=02-22-2013. Last updated February 22, 2013.

"U.S. Horse Industry Statistics." *The Equestrian Channel*. Accessed February 20, 2013, http://www.theequestrianchannel.com/sitebuildercontent/sitebuilderfiles/2002USEFdemographics.pdf.

Viegas, Jennifer. "Horses Never Forget Human Friends." *Science on NBC News*. http://www.nbcnews.com/id/35911274/ns/technology_and_science-science/#.UUDPMhl40sk. Last updated March 17, 2010.

Wallner, Barbara, C. Vogl, P. Shukla, J.P. Burgstaller, T. Druml, et al. "Identification of Genetic Variation on the Horse Y Chromosome and the Tracing of Male Founder Lineages in Modern Breeds." PLoS ONE 8(4): (2013) e60015. doi:10.1371/journal.pone.0060015.

"What is Dressage?" *Equine Canada*. Accessed February 18, 2013,
    http://equinecanada.ca/dressage/index.php?option=com_conten
    t&view=category&id=2&Itemid=545&lang=en
When I Am an Old Horsewoman. Accessed June 25 2013, http://www.
    equinese.com/OldHorsewomanPoem.htm.
Williams, Lisa Ross. "A Natural Approach to Laminitis." *International
    Alliance for Animal Therapy and Healing*. Accessed March 5, 2013,
    http://www.iaath.com/naturalapproachtolaminitis.htm.

Index

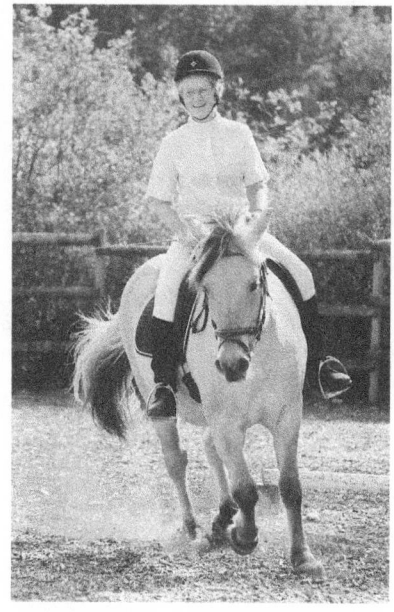

ALICE MACGILLIVRAY IS a leadership consultant, university faculty member, author, wife, and mother. She dreamed of owning a horse as a child but set the dream aside for decades to focus on work and family. In her fifties, she realized it was now or never. Alice lives on Gabriola Island, British Columbia.

ABOVE *The author on her mare Bocina on their first dressage test day.* Photo: BRANDI MEYER

CPSIA information can be obtained
at www.ICGtesting.com
Printed in the USA
BVHW072302241119
564682BV00003B/282/P